INTERPROFESSIONAL EDUCATION IN EUROPE:
POLICY AND PRACTICE

"It takes two flints to make a fire."

— Louisa May Alcott

Every attempt has been made to ensure the accuracy and reliability of the information in this book. Neither the authors nor the publisher can be held responsible for any inconvenience due to possible inaccuracies which readers may encounter in this book.

Andre Vyt, Majda Pahor & Tiina Tervaskanto-Maentausta (eds.)

# Interprofessional education in Europe: Policy and practice

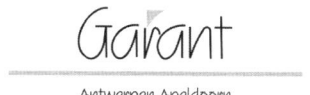

Antwerpen-Apeldoorn

Andre Vyt, Majda Pahor & Tiina Tervaskanto-Maentausta (eds.)
Interprofessional education in Europe: Policy and practice
Antwerpen/Apeldoorn
Garant
2015

126 pages – 24 cm
ISBN 978-90-441-3334-9
D/2015/5779/78
NUR 840

Cover design: Koloriet
Lay-out and graphics: Zatande

© The authors & Garant Publishers nv

All rights protected. Other than exceptions specified by the copyright law,
no part of this publication may be reproduced, stored or made public,
in any way whatsoever, without the express, prior and written permission
of the authors and of the publisher.

*Garant Publishers*
Somersstraat 13-15, 2018 Antwerp, Belgium
www.garant-uitgevers.be – info@garant.be
*Garant Publishers*
Koninginnelaan 96, 7315 EB Apeldoorn, The Netherlands
www.garant-uitgevers.nl – info@garant-uitgevers.nl
Garant/Central Books
99, Wallis Road, London E9 5 LN, Great-Britain
www.centralbooks.com – bill@centralbooks.com
Garant/ISBS
920 NE 58th Ave Suite 300, Portland, OR 9721311, USA
www.isbs.com – info@isbs.com, orders@isbs.com

# Table of contents

| | |
|---|---|
| Contributors | 6 |
| Editorial introduction | 7 |
| Strengthening the links between practice and education in the development of collaborative competence frameworks | 9 |
| Beyond interprofessionalism: Caring *together with* rather than *for* people | 37 |
| Creating spaces for interprofessional learning: Strategic revision of a common IPL curriculum in undergraduate programmes | 49 |
| Interprofessional education in health and social care: Changing students' opinions | 67 |
| The development and implementation of an IP education programme: A multifaceted approach | 77 |
| IPE in undergraduate medical and health care studies: Collaboration with authorities, public services and schools | 91 |
| Focused interprofessional courses: Aiming for effective competence acquisition | 107 |
| Everyone benefits: Interprofessional work placement | 117 |
| Epilogue | 125 |

# Contributors

The following persons have contributed to this volume (listed per country and alphabetically by first name):

Belgium: Andre Vyt (Health Care and Teacher Training Departments of Artevelde University College and Faculty of Medicine and Health Sciences of the University of Ghent), and Bianka Vandaele (Department of Speech Therapy and Audiology of Artevelde University College Ghent).

Finland: Anja Taanila (Faculty of Medicine of the University of Oulu and Unit of Primary Health Care of the University Hospital of Oulu), Essi Varkki (Faculty of Medicine of the University of Oulu), Tiina Tervaskanto-Mäentausta (School of Health of the Oulu University of Applied Sciences and the Faculty of Medicine of the University of Oulu), and Ulla-Maija Seppänen (School of Health of the Oulu University of Applied Sciences).

Netherlands: Albine Moser, Anita Stevens, and Sandra Beurskens (Faculty of Health Care of Zuyd University Heerlen), Ivo Hendriks, Karin van Beek, Marjolein Thijssen, Menno Pistorius, and Wietske Kuijer-Siebelink (Department of Health of HAN University of Applied Sciences Nijmegen).

Sweden: Annika Lindh Falk, Annika Heslyk, Johanna Dahlberg, Madeleine Abrandt Dahlgren, Mattias Ekstedt, and Per Whiss (Faculty of Health Sciences of Linköping University).

Slovenia: Barbara Domajnko, Majda Pahor, Matic Kavčič, Nevenka Ferfila, Renata Vettorazzi, and Teja Škodič Zakšek (Faculty of Health Sciences of the University of Ljubljana).

United Kingdom: Sarah Hean, University of Stavanger (Norway) and Bournemouth University (UK).

The editors wish to thank Marion Helme for proofreading chapters and checking for correct English spelling and phrasing.

# Editorial introduction

Interprofessional education (IPE) is acknowledged as a need in higher education based on societal demands. The impact of interprofessional collaboration on the quality of care and on the quality of human health is substantial. A continuous effort is needed to underpin interprofessional learning and teaching with evidence and to support it with tools created by research and development. We hope that this book encourages other people, professionals as well as academics and policymakers, to engage themselves in fostering the further development of this domain.

IPE itself also needs to be appropriately focused. The definition of interprofessional education as described already at the end of the previous century by the Centre for Advancement in Interprofessional Education (CAIPE) is essential, namely as occasions when two or more professions learn with, from and about each other to improve collaboration and the quality of care. Not a single word in this definition is superfluous. It is clearly different from occasions when two or more professions simply learn side by side for whatever reason.

IPE receives a growing attention from institutions across Europe. During the past thirty years, many initiatives have been undertaken. The *Journal of Interprofessional Care* but also international meetings of *All Together for Better Health* (ATBH) and of *The Network Towards Unity for Health* (TUFH) have strengthened the dissemination of practices and evidence-based underpinnings. IPE has become a global movement, with networks in Europe, Canada, Australia, Japan, and the USA.

The challenge for institutions in Europe to implement IPE may be harder than in other regions, due to the mosaic of countries having each their own legislation on education and health care. Therefore the mission of a European network needs to put IPE in the spotlights without intermission. A series of All Together Better Health Conferences have been hosted on European soil: in 2006 at Imperial College London (UK) by CAIPE, in 2008 in Stockholm by Karolinska Institutet and Linkoping University with the Nordic Interprofessional Network, and in 2016 in Oxford (UK) by CAIPE, the University of Oxford and Oxford Brookes University. The biannual conferences of the European Interprofessional Practice & Education Network (EIPEN) started in 2007, and has been hosted in Poland, Finland, Belgium, Slovenia, and the Netherlands. Country-based foundations, networks of institutions, and professional bodies throughout Europe in the coming years may explicitly acknowledge IPE not simply as an added value but as a necessity for the accreditation of study programmes as well as for professionals in health care.

Following WHO's Framework for Action (2010) already in 2011 EIPEN has adopted a charter stating the synergy between different actors as a condition for effective collaborative practice to become true. This charter stipulates the following requirements (see www.eipen.eu):

- Professional bodies of health and social care professions but also health insurance agencies and patient organisations explicitly formulate the necessity of competences in interprofessional collaboration being present in graduating students in health and social care professions.
- Educational and clinical institutions formulate interprofessional collaborative work as one of the main values in their mission and in their quality management policy, and support and adhere to bodies and networks that promote and/or supervise interprofessional health and social care.
- Higher educational institutions ensure that graduates are competent in interprofessional care and professional body representatives ratify educational programmes based on the presence of interprofessional competences.
- Clinical institutions ensure that staff is competent in interprofessional care, by providing continuous training and by allowing patient representatives and/or representatives from patient organisations to take part in the institutional policy
- Governmental agencies focus on the compliance of clinical and educational institutions with regulations promoting and necessitating interprofessional practice and education, and support the institutions by implementing accreditation and financial mechanisms that foster this practice and education.

Interprofessional collaboration requires transdisciplinary mindsets, instruments and mechanisms (Vyt 2015). Inspiring examples can be helpful. This book may contribute to the development of IPE in higher education institutions where IPE is not yet deployed, but also in institutions where IPE is present but not fully developed. It provides policy issues and examples of good practice, showing elements which have to be taken into account when developing and implementing interprofessional courses, course units, or study programmes.

## Literature

Vyt A (2015). Interprofessional education and collaborative practice in health and social care: The need for transdisciplinary mindsets, instruments and mechanisms. In P Gibbs (Ed.), *Transdisciplinary professional learning and practice* (pp.69-88). Heidelberg/Zug: Springer.

World Health Organisation (2010). *Framework for action on interprofessional education & collaborative practice*. Geneva: WHO.

# Strengthening the links between practice and education in the development of collaborative competence frameworks

Sarah Hean

There is need for greater synergy between practice needs and educational provision, with the education system needing to respond appropriately to current and future population needs. They do so by preparing adequate numbers of professionals with the appropriate skills to be able to provide services that address these needs (Frenk e.a. 2010, IOM 2015).

The advancement of science and technology means care is increasingly complex and specialised. This increase in complexity is partially a response to a rapidly changing health and welfare environment. Innovations are constantly required to find new solutions to these challenges. Innovation competence is therefore a must within health and welfare organisations and educational institutions alike (Frenk e.a. 2010).

Although modern services are highly specialised, population needs are, in contrast, closely interwoven requiring co-ordination of services or activities at a systems level and positive collaborative relations at the professional level. Textbox 1 illustrates this interdependence of needs within a vulnerable population requiring multiple professional and organisational input. Integration and collaboration competencies are required to address this.

Many contemporary challenges in health and welfare are wicked in nature being complex, hard to pin down and define. Every user's problem is unique, multi-dimensional, both unstable and highly interrelated. Solutions are hard to predict and measure and often do not lend themselves to standardised care pathways (Rittel & Webber 1973). Practitioners must be flexible, be able to see the whole picture, be able to deal with uncertainty and the bespoke nature of each service user's health challenges.

Textbox 1: The current needs of the mentally ill offender population as an illustration of contemporary population needs

Mentally ill offenders, as one vulnerable population, have multiple needs in addition to their mental illness including substance misuse, housing, training and financial needs (Sverdrup 2013). An offender, with mental health issues, will require stable, supported living type housing, upon release in order to be able to register for municipal mental health services and cope with their condition in a supported, stable, drug free environment (with drugs often being strongly related to their mental health condition). The psychiatrist's task of mental health treatment is therefore dependent on the prison social worker being able to find suitable housing for the offender. This task is in turn dependent on housing officers in the offender's home community being able to identify and allocate suitable housing stock. This sequential interdependence between tasks may break down if each of these professionals is unable to communicate frequently and in a timely and accurate manner (Gittell 2011) across professional and organisational boundaries, highlighting to each other the offender's needs and the constraints that each service are working under (e.g. lack available housing stock, public safety issues).

---

Add to the melting pot, unacceptably high levels of critical incidents and breaches of client safety due to poor interprofessional collaboration (National Patient Safety Agency 2011) as well as the grey spaces into which clients fall as they make the transitions between highly differentiated and unintegrated health and social care services or from primary to secondary/institutional care (and back again) (Valentijn e.a. 2013). Increased client expectations, fostered in a culture of new public management (Alford 2009) means that there are added pressures from service users that their experiences of these transitions will be positive ones, that professionals are able to communicate and collaborate with each other and the service user themselves and that service leaders are able to design integration models that encourage these behaviours.

Many of the above needs described require a work force that is collaboratively competent (Frenk e.a. 2010). In this chapter we explore collaborative competence, especially the theoretical underpinnings behind these, in greater detail. We position this framework as in fact a central domain in a range of wider but interrelated set of competency frameworks, namely social innovation and integration competencies. We explore also the relevance of theoretical competence, as relevant to all three of the above frameworks.

But, we first define and position competencies ontologically and add some caveats related to an over reliance on such competence based approaches to education.

## Competencies

Fraser & Greenhalgh (2001) define competence as "what individuals know or are able to do in terms of knowledge, skills, and attitude". They differentiate this from capability — "the extent to which individuals can adapt to change, generate new knowledge, and continue to improve their performance" (p. 799). Learners need to develop the ability to integrate knowledge, skills, attitudes and values in making professional judgements and into each new professional experience they encounter (Bainbridge e.a. 2010, Orchard & Bainbridge 2010).

Capability does not develop within a vacuum and will be nurtured in environments that promote collaborative cultures and invest resources in the systems that allow collaboration to happen more efficiently and effectively. Carlile (2004) refers to this added dimension when defining capability as a function of individual ability (or competence) and capacity (external resource). The concept may be viewed therefore both as an individual and organisational feature (Darsø 2012) or alternatively as expertise that lies in both the system and in individuals ability to recognise and negotiate its use (Edwards & Kinti, 2009). For the remains of the chapter, for simplicity we continue to use the term competence but with the understanding that this encompasses the above characteristics of capability.

The emphasis on competency based education is a behaviourist approach to learning, where focus is less on thought processes and how learning has occurred (the focus of constructivist educators). It emphasises learning outcomes (Hean e.a. 2009). Figure 1 positions competency based education in relation to some other educational approaches.

Before exploring relevant competencies that students require, it is essential, in order to strengthen the link between practice and education systems, that competencies are reconnected to the practice behaviours these are intended to encourage. For each competency framework discussed, therefore, I begin with some of the dimensions underpinning the practice behaviour. The competency frameworks should reflect these dimensions. Competency frameworks are largely created through a review of existing competency frameworks (uni- and inter-professional) and literature on existing competency frameworks, single professional body guidelines and interviews with stakeholders. Valid though these consensus building exercises may be, they are strengthened if a clear theory and evidence based rationale, rooted in actual collaborative practice, are provided to defend the inclusion of each domain and if the relationship between domains, the approach to domain design and how these domains are translated into professional practice are explored. I explore how this may or may not have been achieved in some exemplar frameworks.

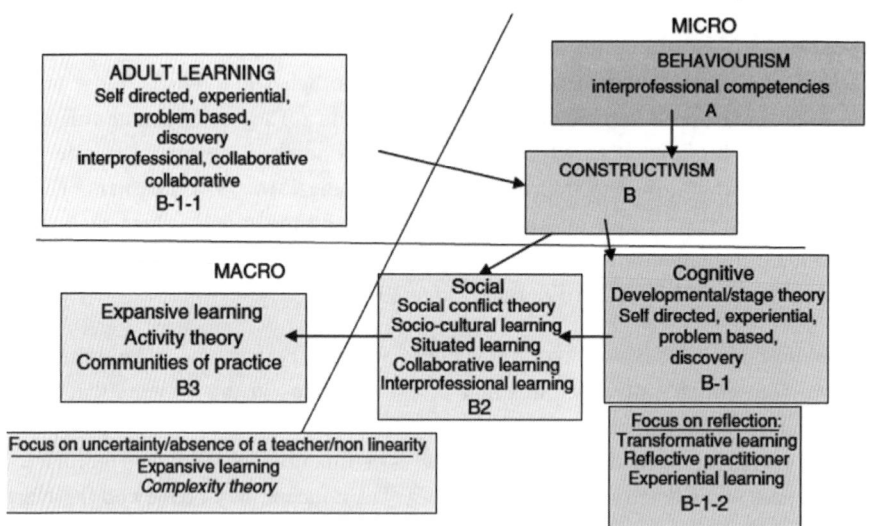

Figure 1: Positioning of competency based approaches in relation to some other educational approaches (Hean e.a. 2009).

## Collaborative competence

Collaborative practice is defined as occurring when multiple health workers from different professional backgrounds provide comprehensive services by working with patients, their families, caregivers and communities to deliver the highest quality of care across settings (World Health Organisation 2010). Collaboration is a multi-dimensional and multilevel construct, captured in the empirically based Perception of Interprofessional Collaboration Model (PINCOM) (Ødegård 2006). Interviews with key practice stakeholders and reviews of collaboration literature identified 12 main concepts under the collaboration umbrella. At an individual level, perceptions of professional power differences between collaborators, clarity in role expectations, personality style and motivation to work in a collaborative way, were identified as key dimensions. At group level, communication between professionals, support received from fellow group members, coping strategies when collaborating team functioning and collaborative leadership were viewed as important. Finally, collaborators often work for a range of organisations with different priorities, with cultures that encourage or discourage collaborative action, where the environment or systems may or may not be in place that allow interactions to flow smoothly and where there is varying clarity about what other organisations do. No theoretical links between domains have been suggested within PINCOM so far and a theoretical model predicting the relationship between different dimensions of collaboration, demographic variables (input) and professional and organisational outcomes (output) is still to be tested (Strype e.a. 2014).

Models exploring the construct of Relational Coordination and its antecedents and influence (Gittell, Seidner & Wimbush 2010) are more advanced in this regard, although fewer key dimensions of collaboration are included and only at the group level. Relational Coordination (RC) is defined as the coordination of work through positive interprofessional relationships (Gittell 2011).

The coordination part is conceived as the frequent, high-quality communication between different professionals (communication that is accurate, timely and leads to problem solving). This in turn is influenced by (and has an influence on) quality relations between professionals, quality assessed in terms of having shared goals, shared/common knowledge of each other's roles, and mutual respect. Empirical testing of the model has shown positive relationships between a variety of system based interventions (e.g. selection for team players in recruitment, interprofessional team meetings etc.) and relational coordination. In so doing it provides a useful link between current political drivers towards structural integration between systems and services and the behaviour of the workforce within these systems (see Figure 2). Relationships between relational coordination and outcomes are also noted. For example relationships are found between re-offending rates in offenders released from prison and the quality of relations between professionals in the criminal justice and community services. The direction of the relationship is not always in the expected direction as significant inverse relationships may mean professionals are brought together in times of crisis (Bond & Gittell 2010).

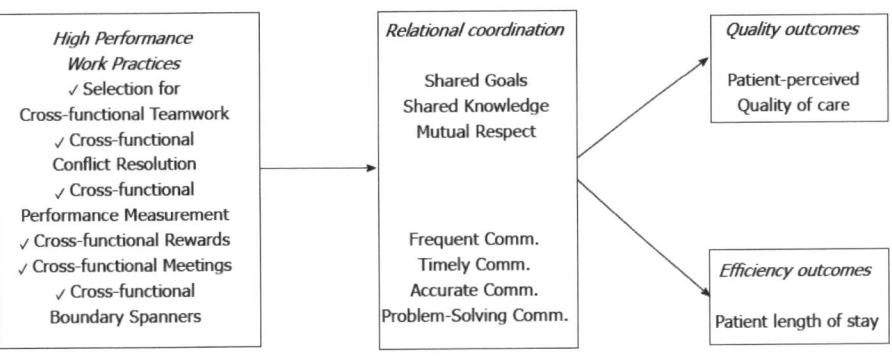

Figure 2: Model exploring relationship between Practices supporting integration, relational coordination and patient and organisational outcomes (Gittell 2011).

It follows that these dimensions of collaboration in practice should be the backbone of collaborative competency frameworks. Some recent examples of such interprofessional competency frameworks are given in Table 1.

Table 1: Examples of collaborative competencies in different models.

| Model | Domains | Exemplar competence |
| --- | --- | --- |
| Metacognitive Interprofessional competencies model (Wilhelmsson e.a. 2012) | Teamwork/group processes<br>Reflection & documentation<br>Communication<br>Shared knowledge<br>Ethics | *Shared knowledge:* Awareness of general laws/rules for all health/social professions. |
| Core competencies for collaborative practice framework (Interprofessional Education Collaborative 2011) | Teams and Teamwork<br>Roles/Responsibilities<br>Communication<br>Values/Ethics | *Roles/Responsibilities:* Communicate one's roles & responsibilities clearly to patients, families, other professionals. |
| National interprofessional competency framework (Orchard & Bainbridge 2010) | Team functioning<br>Communication<br>Patient-centred care<br>Role clarification<br>Conflict resolution<br>Collaborative leadership | *Collaborative leadership:* Co-creation of a climate for shared leadership and collaborative practice. |
| Interprofessional capabilities framework (Walsh e.a. 2012) | Interprofessional working<br>Knowledge in Practice<br>Reflection<br>Ethical Practice | *Interprofessional working:* Able to lead/participate in interprofessional team and wider inter-agency work, to ensure responsive, integrated approach to care/service management focused on the needs of the patient. |

Frenk e.a. (2010) describing trends in instructional design, encourages the move from problem based approaches to learning to this type of competency based education stating that: "By focusing on the outcomes of education, the approach is more transparent and therefore accountable to learners, policy makers, and stakeholders. Metrics and assessment with a wide variety of methods are integral to the competency-based approach, which depends on assessment of progress or shortcomings in achieving competencies" (p. 21).

This is essentially a repopularisation of the behaviourist approach to learning, as described earlier, a move away from constructivist approaches focused on the process of learning (Table 2).

Table 2: Move from problem-based approaches to competency based education (based on Frenk e.a. 2010).

| 20th century | 21st century |
|---|---|
| Experiential/Problem-based learning<br>Constructivist<br>Emphasis on how to learn<br>(self-directed, experiential) | Competency-driven education<br>Behaviourist<br>Outcome based<br>(knowledge, skills and attitudes) |

It could be argued that this approach is already in line with current trends in the broader spheres of curriculum development, other than those focused on collaboration competencies alone, where key learning outcomes are a central part of most contemporary curriculum designs (Biggs & Tang 2007). Behaviourist approaches are indeed already evident in the design and evaluation of interprofessional education programmes that employ the Kirkpatrick model of educational outcomes, for example (e.g. Freeth e.a. 2002, McNair e.a. 2001, Carpenter, Barnes, Dickinson & Wooff 2006).

Such a behaviourist approach is likely to appeal to those more comfortable with a positivist stance in research and curriculum development in which clear outcomes are expected, assessed and evaluated. Such a clear cut, structured approach has its appeal. However, if chosen to underpin an evaluation of collaborative training or curriculum design, it must be acknowledged that, in focusing exclusively on the outcomes or products of learning, the educator ignores the processes that have underpinned this. So where we agree with Frenk e.a. (2010) that an over focus on problem based learning has led to an absence of tangible learning outcomes in these collaborative training programmes, a swing to the other extreme is not desirable either. A focus on competencies and a behaviourist curriculum approach that emphasizes learning by doing, learning by trial and error, and the consequences of one's own behaviour, is in danger of producing students that are over involved in practicalities of experience, and fail to reflect on their actions during this process. Students are in danger of becoming overly focused on the assessment and achieving the stated behavioural objectives (Bigge & Shermis 1999, Armitage e.a. 2003, Hean e.a. 2009). There is a midway, however, taken by two exemplar collaborative competency frameworks (Orchard & Bainbridge 2010, Wilhelmsson e.a. 2012) that combine, in an integrated approach, a competency-based curriculum, with a continued reflection on processes of learning.

First, the National interprofessional competency (NIC) framework (Orchard & Bainbridge 2010) positions each competency domain in relation to the other. The domains of interprofessional communication and patient-centred care are core and relevant to all inter professional situations and with impact on the other four domains of role clarification, team functioning, interprofessional conflict resolution and collaborative leadership, competencies in themselves not always applicable to every situation the student faces (see Figure 3).

The NIC framework makes clear the approach taken to the design of the framework, exploring Roegiers' range of approaches to building competency frameworks (Roegiers 2007). These range from a skills approach that identifies specific skills needed to perform one particular task or role, life-skills approaches about the development of people as citizens, a competency-based focused purely on the outcomes of learning rather than the process (as recommended by Frenk e.a. 2010), and an integrative approach incorporating all of the above where students are encouraged to integrate knowledge, skills, attitudes, and values in making professional judgments and reflect explicitly on the learning process as they do so.

The NIC Framework positions itself in relation to practice by highlighting how the application of each of competence contributes to the formulation of professional judgement and recognises that these competencies are practised within simple (a few professionals) to complex situations (larger more varied teams), and that there is always patient safety and quality improvement at the heart of all of these competencies. There is an understanding that context (e.g. paediatric versus emergency teams) will lead to context specific skills but that the professional will rely on these core competencies when changing environments until new context specific competencies have been developed. Context, quality improvement and complexity underpin the description of each domain (see Figure 3). The 6 domains within the NIC framework reflect the dimensions of collaborative practice described by Ødegård (2006), albeit developed in a different country context and the focus being on education rather than collaborative practice. This synergy between components of collaboration from education versus practice perspectives validates the domains chosen for inclusion in this framework.

Secondly, a metacognitive competency framework (Willhelmson e.a. 2012) also takes an integrated approach to instructional design, combining existing competency framework domains within a metacognitive model where students are able to reflect on their own learning. Although the relationship between domains is not described in this framework, it does, like the NIC model, focus on how competencies relate to professional action or judgement making. In this model (that draws on a previous model of Forslund 2001, see Figure 4).

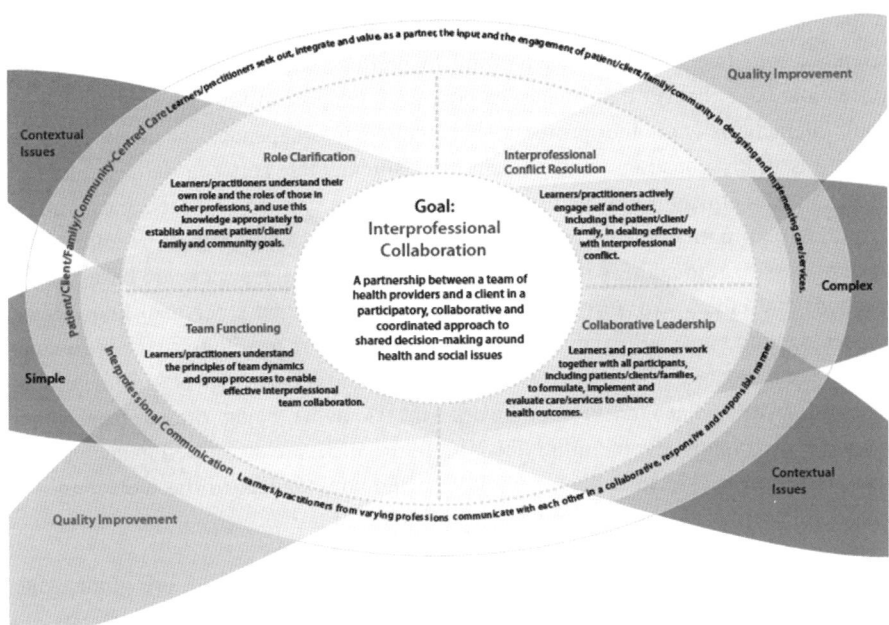

Figure 3: Conceptual model underpinning NIC framework (Orchard & Bainbridge 2010).

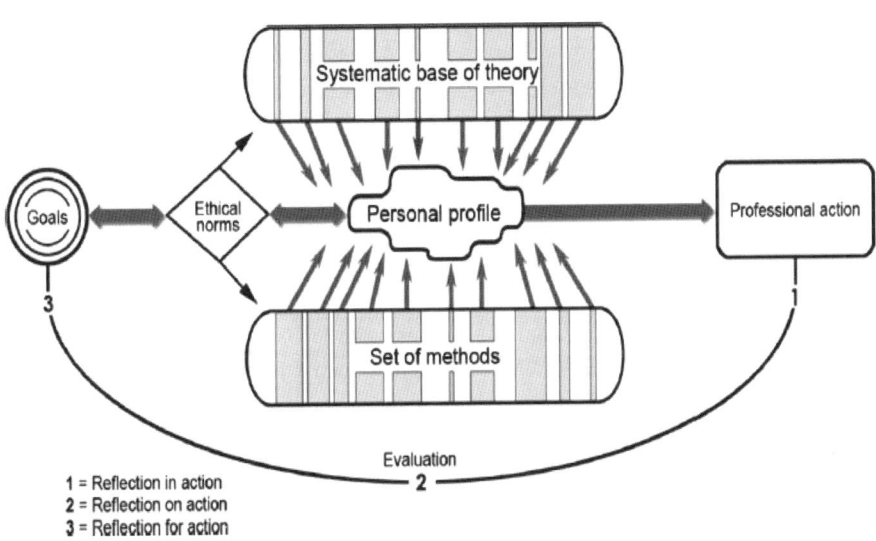

Figure 4: Conceptual framework underpinning the Metacognitive Collaborative Competency framework (Wilhelmsson e.a. 2012).

Wilhelmsson e.a. (2012) propose that work related goals with be informed by the scientific, practice based knowledge and theoretical knowledge (together forming systematic base theory) that underpins how each profession views a certain task or goal. Interactions with other professions to achieve interdependent goals are positive if there is firstly constructive alignment (see Biggs 2003) between the task and the professional's ethical norms and secondly, if professionals share these ethical values or norms (e.g. patient-centredness). Profession-specific methods will be applied by each professional to address the task. The components of the systematic base theory, methods and ethics will all be mediated by each individual's personal knowledge, experience and personality and combine to form a unique profile for each individual professional engaging in any decision making around a particular task. The competencies in the metacognitive framework (the domains being drawn from other competency frameworks including the NIC framework) are structured in such a way that students are able to reflect explicitly on the components of the metacognitive model for each of the competency domains listed (Table 3).

Students do not only think about their own individual profile, but are guided into thinking about how group level profiles (important in interprofessional working) and organisational profiles (important in interorganisational working) develop. This again mirrors Ødegård's (2006) description of individual, group and organisation dimensions of collaboration.

Neither the NIC nor Metacognitive Collaborative Competency frameworks are theories themselves but ways of structuring the description of the skills and competencies students require. Theorisation enters the equation during discussion of how framework designs may improve learning outcomes, in predictions of how domains may interrelate with one another and how the acquisition of competencies might predict practice outcomes such as professional actions, judgements and/or decision making. The NIC model is underpinned by the proposition that professional judgement is a product of the stated competency domains, the practice context and a focus on quality improvement. Similarly, they propose that communication and patient-centred competencies are central components of the four remaining competency domains. Similarly the metacognitive framework sees professional action as mediated by individual factors and profession specific base theories, ethical norms and methods. Both frameworks would be strengthened with testing the propositions put forward or drawing on other pretested theories and the evidence base. The theoretical and evidence base underpinning the inclusion of each domain could be included also by asking, for example, what is the evidence base supporting the link between interprofessional communication in practice and positive outcomes for patients or what are theories that predict and or explain this relationship? Measures of relational coordination between hospital professionals (encompassing the communication domain) are significantly related to patient reports of treatment quality and length of stay (Gittell, Seidner & Wimbush 2010) for example and activity theory and the concept of knotworking are potential theoretical explanations for how communication occurs across these systems (Varpio e.a. 2008).

## Innovation competencies

For many practitioners, however, improving collaboration and relations with other professional groups or organisations are not a priority: there are other constraints, such as financial and manpower resource, and cuts to this, that prevent interorganisational involvement leading to poor patient outcomes. Innovative ways of working across organisations (both bottom up and top down innovation) are required to develop methods in which organisations can work together and positive patient outcomes be achieved despite resource constraint. But collaboration cannot be ignored as interorganisational and interprofessional collaboration and positive relationships are an essential component of this innovation in the first place (Vangen & Huxham 2013, Hean e.a. 2015) .

Innovation requires more than a simple transfer of information between partners but the coproduction of new ways of thinking between them. It requires collaboration through which three main boundaries are transcended. First information must be transferred between partners, it must then be translated into a form all partners can understand and finally transformed into a new product in which the priorities of all partners are accounted for and silo specific political interests compromised (Carlile 2004). This strong link between innovation and collaboration means that collaborative competencies cannot be viewed in isolation and their overlap with social innovation should be considered also.

Innovation (specifically social innovation) is about creating new solutions to effect positive social change, improving social relations and collaborations to address a social demand. It is about taking new knowledge or combining existing knowledge in new ways or applying it to new contexts. Rapidly developing health technologies and increasing complex population needs, as well as demands for greater provision despite dwindling resource, means that there is a continuous drive for innovation in health and welfare, not for competitive advantage but for the advantage of society as a whole (European Commission 2013).

Social innovation has four main elements: *problem identification*: pinpointing new/unmet/inadequately met social needs; *problem solving*: creating new solutions in response to these social needs, *evaluation*: effectiveness of new solutions in meeting social needs and *implementing and scaling up* of effective social innovations (European Commission 2013). Darsø (2012) in distinguishing between the preject and project phases of innovation work, focuses on the problem identification and design of new solution stages, articulating key dimensions in terms of an innovation diamond (Figure 5) in which the concepts of knowledge, ignorance, concepts and relations play a part. Innovation occurs when individuals from different professions or disciplines interact and their profession specific scientific and practice based knowledge is central for any innovation and creativity but it can be limiting if static and dogmatically held by any particular team member. Ignorance is therefore an equally important measure, an openness to identifying and resolving what is not known. This is an uncertain and anxiety laden place to be. Part of innovation is also about developing new concepts, but in developing the new concepts, and critiquing old ones, there needs to be an element of shared under-standing. Words may not be enough to reach this shared understanding and other means of visualising concepts may be required (e.g. prototypes or narratives). The final component of the diamond is the positive relations between participants required for the innovation to take place. There needs to be a movement to and fro between application of existing knowledge and the development of new knowledge and exploration of ignorance, between what is known and not known. Similarly optimum relations between participants will help develop common perceptions of the new concepts and developing innovations. Darsø superimposes onto this model, the leadership roles that are required to manage each of these dimensions within the innovation diamond, with a separate leadership role needed to nurture relations between participants (relations), another to ask those questions that will pinpoint what is not known and stimulate the group to ask questions and propose ideas (ignorance), a third person to encourage the group to describe and illustrate information and knowledge in different ways (concepts) and the final role to establish the current knowledge of participants and the contribution this knowledge makes to the task (knowledge).

The inclusion of the relations dimension within the diamond of innovation model highlights the importance of collaboration to social innovative practice. In fact, social innovation requires a particular kind and depth of collaboration competence although not all forms of collaboration will lead to innovation or this level of co-production style collaboration (Huxom & Vangen 2000, Vangen & Huxham 2013, Hean 2015).

So what competencies are required for the workforce to be socially innovative? Darsø (2012) describes innovation competence as the ability to create innovation by navigating complex processes together with others. This mirrors the call for students to be trained as change agents to transform society (Frenk e.a. 2010). Although Darsø outlines the tasks of key leadership roles (including nurturing relations, creating shared understandings etc.), innovation skills are not required by leadership alone. Leaders, in radical innovation, may plan the redesign of service delivery but innovation can also be more incremental, bricolage, small scale adaptations of practice procedures by frontline professionals, adapting these to each individual client, working within and beyond the constraints systems place upon them (Fuslang 2010). Some of the competencies required for both incremental and radical social innovation are listed in Table 3.

Innovation requires professionals to be reflective and willing to cross organisational and disciplinary borders (Hean e.a. 2015, Huxom & Vangen 2000). Therefore, social innovation competence and collaboration competencies are closely interwoven. In fact collaboration is a key dimension of being innovation competent although the reverse is not always true as not all collaboration will necessary lead to innovation.

Darsø (2012) differentiates between the above individually held innovation competencies and organisational level competencies, the latter being the organisational supports/systems in place that foster innovation. This includes leadership within the organisation that fosters calculated risk taking, interorganisational working etc. Differentiating between organisational and individual competence is applicable for all the competencies described in this chapter.

We present here two exemplar innovation competence frameworks. The conceptual frameworks of Darsø (2012) and Bezzara (2011) are clearly articulated. Firstly, Darsø presents two competencies: social intra and innovation competency, related to skills needed for social interaction and secondly a sensitivity towards others' perspectives and potential contribution. She describes these two domains as highly interdependent. She then superimposes Heron and Reason's (2008) ways of knowing onto the diamond model of innovation arguing that it is the ways of knowing that inform the ways we build competency (see Figure 6). She uses this exercise to then suggest methods with which these competencies may be developed in learners. It is the application of the innovation diamond, a practice model developed empirically through stakeholder interviews, that provides an empirically and practice based model through which different dimensions of the innovation competence can be interlinked. So, for example, to build positive relations required between professionals from different organisations, and simultaneously trying to explore what is not known in an area, learning spaces are required that bring people together in a comfortable space to learn experientially from being in a room with each other and listening to each other's perspectives. New concepts may emerge as individuals work together exploring ideas. Exploring each other's perspectives and the emergence of new concepts can be difficult to articulate at first, however and aesthetic, expressive methods such as art or dance may help common understanding between participants (presentational knowing).

Table 3: Examples of Innovation competency frameworks.

| Model | Domain | Exemplar skills, attitudes and knowledge |
|---|---|---|
| Diamond model of social innovation competencies (Darsø 2012) | Socio-innovative competency | Mastering social skills needed for interaction. |
| | Intra-innovative competency | Consciousness and sensitivity to one's own and others talents, preferences, potential. |
| University of Michigan Model of Innovation competence (2015) | Creativity | Being able to generate a variety of approaches to problem solving. Being able to find a better way to approach problems through synthesizing and reorganising information. |
| | Enterprising | Being able to identify the actual nature and cause of problems and the dynamics that underlie them. Constantly looking for ways that can improve one's organisation. |
| | Integrating Perspectives | Being open to ideas by listening to suggestions from others and to trying new ideas. Being able to collaborate and working with others and seeking the opinions of others to reach a creative solution. |
| | Forecasting | Being able to evaluate long-term consequences and concluding what a change in systems will result in long-term. Being able to evaluate future directions and risks based on current and future strengths, weaknesses, opportunities and threats. |
| | Managing change | Challenging the Status Quo: Willingness to act against the way things have traditionally been done when tradition impedes performance improvements. |
| Bezarra model (Bezarra 2011) | Critical discussion | Being able to engage in critical discussion, learn through criticism, from others, and also from self-criticism and value criticism. |
| | Strategic focus | Being able to Look for the big picture, take a distant perspective on what is close, envision opportunities for innovation. |
| | Confidence in methods | Having a toolbox (frameworks, methods, techniques) that enables them to make innovative interventions, e.g. concept development, visualizing concepts and user experience scenarios. Prototyping, developing strategies for developing and implementing innovations. |
| | Human-centred approach | Focus on the process, not centred on the technology. |

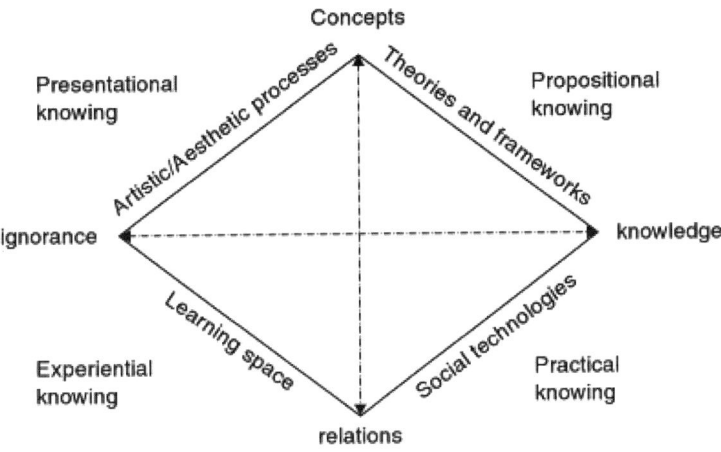

Figure 5: Darsø's (2012) innovation competency diamond.

Knowledge is also built and shared explicitly through words and concepts. In this propositional form of knowing, theoretical models and scientific evidence can be shared between participants (propositional knowing), This enables the knowledge and contribution of participants to be shared. Finally participants will learn by actually doing tasks together (reminiscent of communities of practice described by Wenger (2002) and joint tasks between participants should be planned.

It is difficult to pinpoint the more detailed knowledge, skills, values or attitudes to be developed within the Darsø model (over and above the intra- and social innovation competency described, perhaps because much of the nature of learning will emerge only as the training workshops unfold (see Engeström's (2001) concepts of expansive learning). More detail is provided in the innovation competency framework presented by Bezarra (2011). Bezarra sees innovation in terms of a continuum through which information received from the literature, team members and other sources is retrieved, analysed and synthesised to create shared knowledge.

Through innovation processes this knowledge is converted into a competitive or social advantage. This is made possible through strategic thinking. Finally this advantage is translated into an actually useful product by combining knowledge and strategic thinking into a product or solution to the practice need (see Figure 6). This pathway is matched to the skills required at each phase, providing a framework through which each of these domains can be related to one another. For example research and information gathering skills are required at the beginning of the innovation process (e.g. identification of historical and current trends in the field), followed by analytical skills (e.g. social network analysis of current product/service users). Strategic thinking is required (e.g. conducting a strengths, weaknesses, opportunities and threats analysis and predicting future service requirements) and finally a synthesis phase where ideas and concepts are developed, strategies implemented and communicated.

Key skills throughout this process are the ability to engage on critical discussion, that negates dogmatic profession specific thinking, strategic thinking, that encourages students to take a whole systems view, an ability and confidence to draw on a number of resources and tools that enable research, analysis and synthesis of available resources (including that contained within other members of the innovation team), and lastly a person-centred focus in which innovations have at the forefront the service or product user's needs (the *for who*). The *what* that will be designed as the innovation and how this happens should take second place.

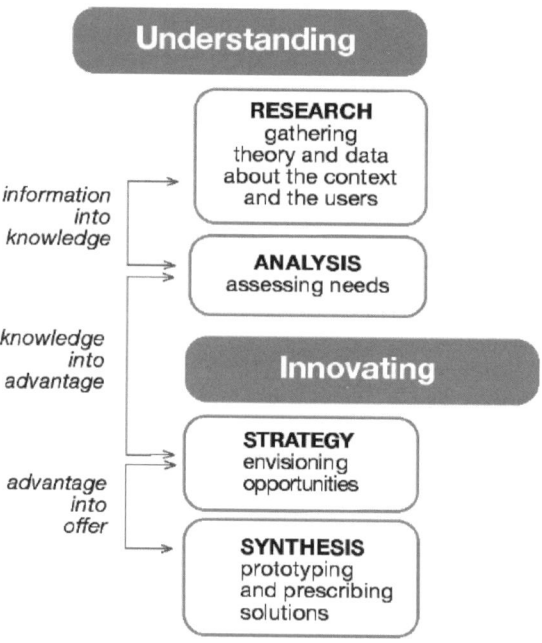

Figure 6: Conceptual model underpinning the innovation competencies model (Bezarra 2011).

Although Bezarra offers a clear and operational competence framework underpinned and held together by a clear conceptual framework, the framework does not report an empirical and practice based underpinning. Further, with the exception of critical discussion skills and communication of the innovation, the relational and potential interdisciplinary aspects of innovation are underplayed in this framework.

## Integration competencies

With the increasing specialisation of services, greater efforts for collaboration between individuals, and integration between services, is required. The importance of this at system level is reflected in the topicality of an integrated care agenda internationally (e.g. World Health Organisation 2015).

Integration is defined by Kodner & Spreeuwenberg (2002) as those methods or models of funding, administration, organisation, service delivery and care designed to create connectivity, alignment and collaboration within and between differentiated sectors with the ultimate aim of enhancing the triple aims (Cerra & Brandt 2011) of quality patient care, experience and service cost-effectiveness. In practice, integration and collaboration agendas have run somewhat in parallel, with integration agenda focusing on the system level and structures that deliver seamless, integrated care and the collaboration field focusing on the relational aspects of inter professional and interorganisational working. Collaboration and integration are in fact different sides of the same coin, each sitting on different ends of the structure versus agency divide, but with models of integration between services facilitating (or constraining) the collaborative behaviour of agents working within these structures.

The models or methods that promote service/organisational integration lie on a continuum from full segregation to full integration, with linkage, coordination and cooperation being intermediate levels between the two extremes. The continuum is not hierarchical and an optimal level of integration between services, will sit somewhere along this continuum dependent on context (Ahgren & Axelsson 2005). The levels of integration can coincide with specific integration devices (Lawrence & Lorsch 1967). For example, at a lesser level of integration, linkage takes place between existing organisational units and relies on timely referral systems moving patients to appropriate services either vertically (between primary and secondary care) or horizontally (between primary care services). Coordination on the other hand, lies further along the integration continuum and is linked to the presence of chains of care or clinical pathways that standardise the procedures, timing and professional input required. Cooperation may involve defined network managers linking the work of independent units at a systems level (Ahgren & Axelsson 2005). Where Ahgren and Axelsson focus on the integration devices along the integration continuum, organisations such as the Centre for Integrated Health Solutions see integration as more geographical in nature (www.integration.samhsa.gov/resource/standard-framework-for-levels-of-integrated-healthcare). The advantage of this continuum is the attempt to link types of integration with collaborative behaviours. The continuum therefore ranges from services being in separately located facilities in which collaboration is minimal or at a distance, to being based in the same facility but in different offices, where basic onsite collaboration may take place, to fully integrated services where services occupy the same geographical space and collaboration is described as being transformed, fully integrated practices, driven by shared concepts and frequent communication. A similar continuum of collaboration is required at the level of knowledge exchange that occurs during collaboration: from simple knowledge transfer to coproduction, which can be mapped against the integration continuum to better understand the level of collaboration each level of integration might engender.

Large scale European initiatives to move integration agendas forward (INTEGRATE, Maturity model of Integration, AQUA) have identified key features to monitor during implementing integration interventions. These dimensions include leadership to drive integration forward with a clear vision on the need and form or degree of integration that will take place, clear structures and governance being in place to support this vision, the development of culture that favours integration and hence stakeholder support (both staff and service user/carer) and removes potential inhibitors whilst promoting facilitators of integration. Integration interventions need to take into account financial and contractual mechanisms and implement information and IT-systems that promote effective information transfer across the integrating units. Evaluation plans should be in place to monitor the outcome of integration models and lastly attention to the preparation of the workforce for integration should be considered (Crawford 2014, AQUA 2015, INTEGRATE 2015). It is this latter preparation of the workforce dimension that is of most relevance to this chapter. Although the focus currently is on processes related to organisational change, there have been attempts to highlight some of the competencies staff need to deliver integrated care (see Hoge e.a. 2014, Table 4).

Hoge e.a. (2014) derived their domains empirically from interviews with key stakeholders and review of the integration literature but apart from reference to the conceptual framework describing the continuum of integration by the Centre for Integrated Solutions, there is no clear theoretical framework that underpins the choice of domains or the relationship between them. Collaboration competencies form a subset of the integration competencies presented in this framework (e.g. interpersonal communications, collaboration and teamwork and cultural competence and adaptation competencies), although no attempt has been made explicitly to distinguish integration from collaboration as concepts within this framework.

There are additional domains that extend beyond collaboration competency frameworks that taking a systems based and more structural view of care (skills related to care planning and coordination, designing interventions with multiple service and organisational input and working within IT-systems that cross service and organisational boundaries). These match some of the key dimensions of integration spelt out in practice by AQUA, Crawford (2014) and INTEGRATE which gives practice based validity to the framework.

Table 4: Integration competencies (Hoge e.a. 2014).

| Domain | Description | Exemplar competence |
|---|---|---|
| INTERPERSONAL COMMUNICATION | Establish rapport quickly and to communicate effectively patients, other professionals etc. | Active listening; conveying information in a jargon-free, non-judgmental manner; using terminology common to the setting in which care is delivered; and adapting to the preferred mode of communication of the consumers and families served. |
| COLLABORATION & TEAMWORK | Function effectively as a member of an inter-professional team including patient. | E.g. understanding and valuing the roles and responsibilities of other team members, expressing professional opinions and resolving differences of opinion quickly, providing and seeking consultation, and fostering shared decision-making. |
| SCREENING & ASSESSMENT | Conduct brief, evidence-based and developmentally appropriate screening and to conduct or arrange for more detailed assessments. | E.g. screening and assessment for: risky, harmful or dependent use of substances; cognitive impairment; mental health problems; behaviors that compromise health; harm to self or others; and abuse, neglect, and domestic violence. |
| CARE PLANNING & CARE COORDINATION | Create and implement integrated care plans. | assisting in the development of care plans, ensuring access to an array of linked services, and the exchange of information between patients and providers, |
| INTERVENTION | Provide a range of brief, focused prevention, treatment and recovery services, longer-term treatment and support for consumers with persistent illnesses. | E.g. motivational interventions, health promotion and wellness services, health education, crisis intervention, brief treatments for mental health and substance use problems, and medication assisted treatments. |
| CULTURAL COMPETENCE & ADAPTATION | Provide services relevant to the culture of patient and family. | Addressing disparities in healthcare access and quality, adapting services to language preferences and cultural norms. |
| SYSTEMS ORIENTED | Function effectively within the organisational and financial structures of healthcare. | E.g. understanding healthcare benefits, or insurances. |
| PRACTICE-BASED LEARNING AND QUALITY IMPROVEMENT | Assess and continually improve the services delivered as an individual provider and as an interprofessional team. | E.g. identifying and implementing evidence-based practices, assessing treatment fidelity, measuring consumer satisfaction and healthcare outcomes, recognizing and rapidly addressing errors in care, and collaborating with other team members on service improvement. |
| INFORMATICS | Use information technology to support and improve integrated healthcare. | E.g. using electronic health records efficiently and effectively; employing computer and web-based screening, assessment, and intervention tools; utilizing telehealth applications; and safeguarding privacy and confidentiality. |

At a practice level, there is overlap also between integration and innovation as concepts as the design and implementation of new models of service integration is a specific area of innovation itself, and as such an area where problem identification, designing new creative solutions, evaluation implementation (and generally managing organisational change) is required. The workforce needs not only to be able to function within established integrated systems but be able to develop new ways in which optimum levels of integration can be achieved in the future. The practice based learning and quality improvement domain of the integration framework, presented in Table 4, best captures the overlap between innovation and integration competency frameworks therefore.

We have found that whilst competency frameworks may be derived from reviews of literature and stakeholder interviews, there is some variation in the degree to which the inclusion of domains in the framework, the relationships between domains and the expected impact that theses competencies have on practice have been theorised. This leads us to a final and related competence, that of theoretical competence.

## Theoretical competence

Theory is a set of propositions/hypotheses linked by a rational argument (Jary & Jary 1995). Underpinning practice is important as theory helps us articulate, reflect and potentially reinterpret our existing/habitual practices. Theory is a tool with which to engage in second-order reflection in which we can stand outside of ourselves looking in on our daily practices with a critical eye (Wackerhausen 2009).

There are a plethora of theories that are on offer that may help us reflect, develop and improve our practices whether this be in the way we think about social innovation, how we consider the design or our work within integrated systems or the collaborative practices required to achieve these. Theories can be drawn from a number of academic disciplines, including sociology, psychology, education and management. The key is to select a theory for its ability to articulate or improve understanding, or rationalise our practice in a particular context. (Kitto e.a. 2011, Hean e.a. 2012, Helme, Jones & Colyer 2005). So, for example, for the clinical practitioner, theory might underpin the strategies they employ to work with other professionals in their work team or transfer information from one organisation to another. For educators, theories on how learning takes place can underpin the interprofessional learning activity. For researchers, theory should underpin the variables selected in the evaluation of an interprofessional programme.

There will also be some element of personal preference when we choose one theory over another. As Wilhelmsson e.a. (2012) state when "choosing theories and methods for future professional work, one's personality and previous knowledge and experiences are intrinsic factors crucial for the kinds of theories and methods that will tend to attract attention and be accepted and integrated in one's emerging professional identity" (p. 87). But whichever theory we choose, it is important that theory is rigorously applied, that we have a clear rationale for practising in a particular way.

A prototype theoretical competency framework has developed through the practice based experiences of the IN-2-THEORY community of practice team (Hean, Anderson e.a. 2012, Hean e.a. in press), consultation with the literature on theory (Fawcett 2005, Fawcett & Downs 1992) and iteratively during a series of workshops aimed at building theoretical competencies (Hean e.a. in press). The framework proposes a range of theoretical competencies, some of the key domains and competences (Table 5).

The means in which theoretical competencies are developed in learners pedagogically is underpinned by the concept of co-creation and the formation of new domains of knowledge when theoretical and practice knowledge overlap during knowledge exchange activities between theorists and professionals (Hammick 1998, Alford 2009, Bernstein 1971). Further, professional narratives are theorised as boundary objects (Carlile 2004) that facilitate the transfer, translation and transformation of knowledge between theorists and professionals in workshops aimed at fostering theoretical competence in professional practice. However, a theoretical underpinning and an empirical underpinning for the choice of each domain as well as the relationship between domains is so far missing and in need of development.

Theoretical competence is already alluded to in the description of collaboration and social innovation competences. Bezarra (2011) for example describes the utility of exploring the theoretical underpinnings of social innovation explicitly with students in their training and Darsø (2012) presents, in her innovation triangle, propositional knowledge (knowledge that is articulated in language) recommending sharing of disciplinary specific theories, in such a way that shared understanding can be achieved. In collaborative competency frameworks, Wilhelmson e.a. (2012) describe the interaction of systematic base theory with ethics and individual characteristics to develop individual, professional and organisational profiles that influence professional decision making. Profession specific scientific theory may be part of the systematic base added to the developing profile (see Figure 6). These must be clearly and precisely communicated to other professions during interprofessional collaborations.

Table 5: Theoretical competencies (Hean e.a. in press).

| Domain | Individual competencies |
| --- | --- |
| APPRECIATION OF THEORY (attitude and knowledge) | Understanding of the importance of theory to rigorous research and practice.<br>Understanding that social meaning of an experience is transformed depending on the theory being applied.<br>Understanding that practice problems have multiple levels and theories can be applied to each of these. |
| KNOWLEDGE OF RELEVANT THEORY (knowledge and skill) | Knowledge of a range of relevant theory applicable to context.<br>Ability to choose a relevant theories from a range of theoretical constructs.<br>Ability to Articulate the key characteristic of the theory chosen, its origins/history (e.g. sociology /psychology) and these historical slants this brings to the one own narrative. |
| APPLICATION OF THEORY (skill) | Use or develop theory to explain why a chosen practice is expected to work and in what context (Pawson & Tilley 2004).<br>Ability to select and apply a relevant theory to a range of different contexts to make alternative meaning of a single experience and hence to aid reflection and decision making in one's practice.<br>Use theory as a reflective tool to either resolve or advance thinking on a range of practice experiences. |
| THEORETICAL QUALITY (skill) | Articulate theory in an accessible manner tailored for the receiving audience.<br>Ensure theory has clear pragmatic value in explaining or predicting a component of practice.<br>Create clear propositions regarding a dimension(s) of practice clearly derived from a chosen theory.<br>Test the theory in practice using appropriate methods. |

In the same way that Wilhelmson e.a. (2012) have introduced a metacognitive element to their collaborative competency frameworks (learners think about learning as they learn), so too would we recommend a metatheoretical approach in which we think about how we theorise, as we theorise and rationalise our actions, with the assumption that this will improve the theoretical rigour of our practice. When developing or applying a competency framework, we need to answer the questions: Why do we expect these specific competency domains to prepare the workforce to address future population demands? Do learners acquire the required competence, and if so how and why? Do they transfer these to the workplace? Is the workplace competent enough itself to allow this transfer and finally, if organisational and individual competence is aligned, are population needs addressed as a result?

We need to predict why and how this pathway takes place and test these theories or alternatively develop rigorous new theory from empirical evidence that also provides these explanations. Anyone involved in educational impact research or evaluation, will understand this is a tall order, bearing in mind the numerous confounding variables that interfere in this pathway, but the intention needs to be there at least, as we struggle to resolve this challenge. Theoretical competence will assist in this task.

The theoretical quality domain spells out the importance of communicating clearly and concisely the meaning of a theory to partners and to articulate explicitly the rationale behind professional decisions making. This has clear application to the social innovation, integration and collaboration frameworks already described. Theoretical competence is required in the future development of these competency frameworks, especially with regard to the domain of theoretical quality. In other words, the theory underpinning the design or delivery or predicted impact of any competency framework should be clearly and concisely articulated to engage the relevant audience. In the evaluation of the competency framework, clear propositions should be created from this theory that can then be tested empirically.

## Conclusions

Collaborative competence is required in the workforce to address current and future population health and welfare needs. Whilst collaborative competence is important in professionals, it should be viewed as connected to other competency frameworks, such as social innovation and integration competence frameworks in which collaboration is a key component. Collaboration competencies are intrinsic to both social innovation and integration competence frameworks. It should be acknowledged however that not all collaboration will lead to innovation, and that a particular depth of collaboration competence is required to develop social innovations. Students need expertise in coproduction that go beyond the ability to simply transfer information frequently in a timely, accurate way (Gittell 2010). Collaboration competencies are also a core relational competence within the integration competence framework but collaborative competencies may be a product of integration competence as well, as well functioning integrated systems should promote positive relations and collaboration within the workforce working within these systems. By linking collaborative competence to other frameworks, the relevance of collaborative competencies to the wider health and care practice arena will be strengthened for both students and practitioners. Similarly, the detail provided in existing collaborative competence frameworks adds to the rigour of the innovation and integration competency frameworks where this dimension may have received less attention.

For all competency frameworks described, this chapter supports the use of an integrated approach to competency development in which both the outcomes and processes of learning are articulated in the framework. Further competence cannot be viewed at an individual level alone and the development of collaboration, innovation and integration competence of the professional, the group and the organisation need all be considered if workforce competence is to have an impact on practice.

I have attempted to reconnect competency domains to practice by considering collaborative, innovation and integration practice in parallel to collaborative, innovation and integration competence frameworks. There was overlap between constructs in the practice and education fields, but at times framework developers referred to existing competency frameworks and interviewing stakeholders about required competencies in their field, rather than maintaining a focus on the evidence or theory from practice. This was more the case in collaborative competency frameworks than integration and innovation spheres. This chapter recommends the evidence based and theoretical underpinnings derived from integration, collaboration and innovation practice arena be consistently introduced into the design of competency frameworks.

There is some variation in the theoretical underpinnings of the frameworks described in this chapter. Whilst not theories themselves, competency frameworks should be underpinned by theory that provides an explanation or predicts how the domains are related, how they are effectively developed in the learner and how these are expected to have an impact on practice. These propositions need to be tested or alternatively supported by practice based empirical evidence elsewhere in the literature. Theoretical competence is also required by front line staff and learners to communicate effectively their profession specific and scientific theories in an effective manner and to reflect on, evaluate and improve their work practices.

## Acknowledgements

This chapter was written with support of funding by the EU Commission FP7 Marie Curie Intra-European Fellowship scheme.

## Literature

Ahgren B & Axelsson R (2005). Evaluating integrated health care: A model for measurement. International *Journal of Integrated Care, 5*, Aug, e01, discussion e03-e09.

Alford J (2009). *Engaging public sector clients*. Basingstoke: Palgrave.

Armitage A, Bryant R, Dunhill R, Renwick M, Hayes D, Hudson A, Kent J & Lawes S (2003). *Teaching and training in post-compulsory education* (2nd edn.). Buckingham: Open University Press.

Advancing Quality Alliance (AQUA) (2015). *Systems Integration Toolkit.* Available at https://www.aquanw.nhs.uk/Downloads/Integrated%20care/System_Integration_Improvement_Resources.pdf.

Bainbridge L, Nasmith L, Orchard C & Wood V (2010). Competencies for interprofessional collaboration. *Journal of Physical Therapy Education, 24* (1), 6–11.

Bernstein B (1971). *Class, codes and control.* London: Routledge.

Bezarra C (2011). *Building innovation capacity.* Otago: University of Otago.

Biggs J (2003). *Teaching for quality learning at university* (2nd edn.). London: Open University Press.

Biggs J & Tang C (2007). *Teaching for quality learning at university.* Maidenhead: Open University Press/McGraw Hill.

Bigge ML & Shermis SS (1999). *Learning theories for teachers* (6th edn.). New York: Longman.

Bond BJ & Gittell JH (2010). Cross-agency coordination of offender reentry: Testing collaboration outcomes. *Journal of Criminal Justice, 38* (2), 118–129.

Carlile PR (2004). Transferring, translating, and transforming: An integrative framework for managing knowledge across boundaries. *Organization Science, 15* (5), 555–568.

Carpenter J, Barnes D, Dickinson, C & Wooff D (2006). Outcomes of interprofessional education for Community Mental Health Services in England: The longitudinal evaluation of a postgraduate programme. *Journal of Interprofessional Care, 20* (2), 145–161.

Cerra F & Brandt BF (2011). Renewed focus in the United States links interprofessional education with redesigning health care. *Journal of Interprofessional Care, 25,* 6, 394–396.

Crawford J (2014). EIP Active & Healthy Ageing B3 – Integrated Care, EHTEL 2014 Symposium, 25-26 November, Brussels. Retrieved March 2015, Available at: http://www.ehtel.eu/references-files/ehtel-2014-symposium-innovating-for-better-outcomes/

Darsø L (2012). Innovation competency: An organisational asset. In S Høyrup, M Bonnafous-Boucher, C Hasse, M Lotz & K Møller (eds), *Employee-Driven Innovation: A new approach.* Basingstoke, UK: Palgrave Macmillan.

Edwards A & Kinti I (2009). Working relationally at organisational boundaries: Negotiating expertise and identity. In H Daniels, A Edwards, Y Engeström & S Ludvigsen (Eds.), *Activity theory in practice: Promoting learning across boundaries and agencies.* London: Routledge.

Engeström Y (2001). Expansive learning at work: Toward an activity theoretical reconceptualization. *Journal of Education and Work, 14* (1), 133–156.

European Commission (2013). *Guide to social innovation.* Brussels: EC.

Fawcett J (2005). Criteria for evaluation of theory. *Nursing Science Quarterly, 18* (2), 131–5.

Fawcett J & Downs FS (1992). *The relationship of theory and research.* Philadelphia: Davis.

Forslund K (2001). Development of professional competence. Department of Pedagogy and Physiology, Linkoping University, Sweden.

Fuglsang L (2010). Bricolage and invisible innovation in public service innovation. *Journal of Innovation Economics, 1* (5), 67-87.

Fraser SW & Greenhalgh T (2001). Coping with complexity: Educating for capability. *British Medical Journal, 323* (7316), 799–803.

Freeth D, Hammick M, Koppel I, Reeves S & Barr H (2002). *A Critical review of evaluations of interprofessional education.* London: LTSN-Centre for Health Sciences and Practices.

Frenk, J, Chen L, Bhutta, Z, Cohen, J, Crisp N, Evans T, Fineberg H, Garcia P, Ke Y, Kelley P, Kistnasamy B, Meleis A, Naylor D, Pablos-Mendez A, Reddy S, Scrimshaw S, Sepulveda J, Serwadda D & Zurayk H (2010). Health professionals for a new century: Transforming education to strengthen health systems in an interdependent world. *Lancet, 376* (9756), 1923–58.

Gittell, JH (2011). Relational Coordination: Guidelines for Theory, Measurement and Analysis. rcrc.brandeis.edu/downloads/Relational_Coordination_Guidelines_8-25-11.pdf

Gittell, JH, Seidner, R & Wimbush, J (2010). A Relational Model of How High-Performance Work Systems Work. *Organization Science, 21*, June, 490–506.

Hean S, Anderson E, Bainbridge L, Clark PG, Craddock D, Doucet S, Hammick M, Mpofu R, O'Halloran C, Pitt R, Oandasan I, Craddock D & Halloran CO (2013). IN-2-THEORY – Interprofessional theory, scholarship and collaboration: A community of practice. *Journal of Interprofessional Care, 27*, 88-90.

Hean, S, Craddock D & Hammick M (2012). Theoretical insights into interprofessional education: AMEE Guide No. 62. *Medical Teacher, 34* (2), e78–101.

Hean S, Craddock D, & O'Halloran C (2009). Learning theories and interprofessional education: A users guide. *Learning in Health and Social Care, 8* (4), 250–262.

Hean S, Doucet S, Bainbridge L, Ball V, Anderson L, Baldwin C, Green C, Pitt C, Snyman S, Schmidtt M, Clark P, Gilbert J, & Oandasan I. (in press). Moving from atheoretical to theoretical approaches to interprofessional client-centred collaborative practice. In C Orchard, C Herbert & L Bainbridge (Eds.), *Interprofessional client-centred collaborative practice – What does it look like? How can it be achieved?* New York: NOVA

Helme M, Jones I & Colyer H (2005). *The theory-practice relationship in interprofessional education.* London: HSAP Subject Centre.

Heron P & Reason J (2008). Extending epistemology within a cooperative inquiry. In P Reason & H Bradbury (Eds.), *Handbook of action research: Participative inquiry and practice.* London: Sage.

Hoge MA, Morris JA, Laraia M, Pomerantz A & Farley T (2014). *Core competencies for integrated behavioral health and primary care.* Washington, DC: SAMHSA - HRSA Center for Integrated Health Solutions.

Huxom C & Vangen S (2000). Leadership in the shaping and implementation of collaborative agendas: How things happen in a (not quite) joined up world. *Academy of Management Journal, 43*, 1159–1175.

Interprofessional Education Collaborative (2011). *Core competencies for interprofessional collaborative practice.* Washington, D.C: Interprofessional Education Collaborative.

Jary DJ & Jary J (1995). *Collins dictionary of sociology.* Glasgow: Collins.

Kitto S, Chesters J, Thistlethwaite J & Reeves S (2011). *Sociology of interprofessional health care practice: Critical reflections and concrete solutions.* New York: NOVA.

Kodner D & Spreeuwenberg LC 2002. Integrated care: Meaning, logic, applications, and implications. *International Journal of Integrated Care, 2*, November, 1–6.

Lawrence PR & Lorsch JW (1967). Differentiation and integration in complex organizations. *Administrative Science Quarterly, 12*, 1-47.

Hammick M (1998). Interprofessional education: Concept, theory and application. *Journal of Interprofessional Care, 12*, 323–332.

McNair R, Brown R, Stone N, Sims JS (2001). Rural interprofessional education: Promoting teamwork in primary health care education and practice. *The Australian Journal of Rural Health, 9*, Suppl 1, S19–26.

Institute of Medicine (2015). *Measuring the impact of interprofessional education on collaborative practice and patient outcomes*. Washington: IOM.

National Patient Safety Agency (2011). *Patient Safety First: The campaign review*. London: National Patient Safety Agency.

Ødegård A (2006). Exploring perceptions of interprofessional collaboration in child mental health care. *International Journal of Integrated Care, 6*, December, e25.

Orchard CA & Bainbridge LA (2010). *A national interprofessional competency framework*. Vancouver: Canadian Interprofessional Health Collaborative.

Project INTEGRATE (2015). Available at http://projectintegrate.eu

Roegiers X (2007). Curricular reforms guide schools: but, where to? *Prospects, 37* (2), 155-186.

Rittel HWJ & Webber M (1973). Dilemmas in a general theory of planning. *Policy Sciences, 4*, 155-169.

Strype J, Gundhus HOI, Egge M & Ødegård A (2014). Perceptions of Interprofessional Collaboration. *Journal of Integrated Care 14*.

Sverdrup S (2013). Evaluering av tilbakeføringskoordinatorene: Analyse av implementerings-prosessen. Unpublished report.

University of Michigan (2015). University of Michigan Model of innovation competence, Available at http://www.umich.edu/~dsafinhr/competencies.html, Retrieved March 2015.

Valentijn PP (2013). Understanding integrated care: A comprehensive conceptual framework based on the integrative functions of primary care. *Journal of Integrated Care, 13*.

Vangen S & Huxham C (2013). Building and using the theory of collaborative advantage. In R Keast, M Mandell & R Agranoff (Eds.), *Network Theory in the Public Sector: Building New Theoretical Frameworks*. New York, NY: Taylor & Francis.

Varpio L, Hall P, Lingard L & Schryer CF (2008). Interprofessional communication and medical error: A reframing of research questions and approaches. *Academic Medicine : Journal of the Association of American Medical Colleges, 83* (10), S76–S81.

Wackerhausen S (2009). Collaboration, professional identity and reflection across boundaries. *Journal of Interprofessional Care, 23*, 455–473.

Walsh M & van Soeren M (2012). Interprofessional learning and virtual communities: An opportunity for the future. *Journal of Interprofessional Care, 26*, 43–48.

Wenger E (2002). Cultivating communities of practice practice: A quick start-up guide. Unpublished document.

Wilhelmsson M, Pelling S, Uhlin L, Lars OD, Faresjo T & Forslund K (2012). How to think about interprofessional competence: A metacognitive model. *Journal of Interprofessional Care, 26*, 85–91.

World Health Organisation (2010). *Framework for action on interprofessional education & collaborative practice*. Geneva: WHO.

World Health Organisation (2015). *Global strategy on people-centred and integrated health services*. Geneva: WHO.

For information on interprofessional practice and education in Europe, visit the website of the European Interprofessional Practice and Education Network (EIPEN):

www.eipen.eu

# Beyond interprofessionalism: Caring *together with* rather than *for* people

Barbara Domajnko, Nevenka Ferfila, Matic Kavčič and Majda Pahor

## Patient involvement in interprofessional education and practice

Designing an interprofessional course is a multifaceted challenge. Among other things, it involves a specific approach to a health care team and collaborative practice. From a sociological perspective, it is important to focus on who is considered to be a member of a health care team and what power relations are established among the team members in their joint activities.

This issue became relevant in surveying the students' knowledge upon entering an interprofessional course for undergraduates in health and social care at the Faculty of Health Sciences of the University of Ljubljana, Slovenia. The elective course brought together final year students from nursing, midwifery, occupational therapy, sanitary engineering, radiography, physiotherapy, as well as medicine, social work and psychology. In 2011-12, the following question was posed to students: "In your opinion, what does interprofessional collaboration mean?" To our surprise, none of the answers mentioned patients as being actively involved. From 2012-13 onward, we phrased the question somewhat differently: "In your opinion, what does collaborative practice in health care mean?" The response changed slightly but promisingly. Sometimes, active collaboration was recognized as a two-level process, also including the patient:

> "It means the collaboration of the patient with a health care team and the collaboration of the health care team members among themselves and with the patient."

Although they may be 'collaborating', the patient was still not considered to be on the team. However, a few students explicitly described collaboration as partnership between professionals, patients and their significant others:

> "The collaboration of all health professionals and the patient in the process of treatment."

*"Collaboration between all the experts involved in the care of a patient, mutual respect, help, counselling; and also the inclusion of the patient in the process and the possibility for them to make decisions about their healthcare."*

*"Co-creation of solutions for the user; it is about communication and goal achievement with joint efforts, among the user and all professionals included in the process of health care and the user's significant others (e.g. relatives)."*

*"In my opinion, collaboration in health care means that I regularly collaborate with the patient to coordinate their needs, wishes, and difficulties. I collaborate with the patient, as well as with all health workers necessary for the patient's recovery and well-being."*

*"For me, it means that all members of the team including the patient collaborate in the process of health care and that they all strive for the improvement of the health care given and complement one another."*

*"Helping others. Collaboration with the patient, other experts to achieve better health."*

We believed this shift in focus was enabled by omitting the word interprofessional from the question, which seemed to indicate strongly that respondents only think about the team/collaboration within the framework of professions and the relations between them. With interprofessional collaboration in mind, a health care team was predominantly defined as being constituted by different health (and health-related) professionals. The interpretation of health care was marked by a patronizing attitude: professionals providing treatment, delivering service, helping and contributing to good outcomes:

*"Networking of different professional in the treatment of the patient."*

*"For me it means that a health care expert expresses his views, opinions and suggestions within the process of health care treatment of a patient (each expert from his own professional field)."*

Professional collaboration was interpreted as being done in the name and for the benefit of the patient's health but according to professionals' best expert knowledge and judgement:

*"Integration of different health care experts in the care of the patient. Everyone works for the benefit of the patient with his or her knowledge. Two heads are better than one."*

> *"Collaboration among experts of different professions who treat the patient and complement their knowledge for his good."*
>
> *"Communication with other members of the team, collaboration and achievement of the common goal by uniting power and knowledge. In this way, the patient is treated in a holistic way, which is also better for them and for their health."*

Patients were understood as people in need of expertise, recipients of professional services, (passive) recipients of what professionals assumed and believed was best ("holistic" and "patient-centred") care for them. Patients were not positioned as partners; there was a clear absence of their voice.

> *"Interprofessional means collaboration of all different health professions in the process of the health care treatment of the patient. Health professionals exchange opinions and together choose the most efficient method of treatment."*
>
> *"It means collaboration of different health professionals with a common goal – to achieve health for the patient."*

At first, our focus was directed towards investigating students' perspectives. Turning to the widely used professional interpretations and definitions, it soon became evident that published views on interprofessional collaborative care are also neither unequivocal nor clear concerning patients as members of their health care team. Patient involvement was addressed differently, or implicit, or missing.

## Can lay people be on the health care team?

The term 'patient-centred care' is widely used in current health profession literature. Gachoud e.a. (2012) found it to be a rather fuzzy container concept. In an interpretive phenomenological study of the interpretation of patient-centredness by members of three professional groups (medicine, nursing and social work) they identified a shared core meaning: identifying, understanding and answering patient's needs. All participants agreed on the importance of an holistic approach and good communication skills. However, is the patient involved in their care or is care done by professionals to the patient, for the patient's benefit? Care can be designed to address the patient's needs, but not necessarily from the patient's perspective. Other dimensions of the concept were found to be more specific to a certain profession: autonomy and empowerment to social work, rapport with the patient to nursing. Researchers identified a hierarchy of patient-centredness, medicine being at the bottom, the least patient-centred (as a consequence of being disease-oriented and evidence-based). Patient-centredness, therefore, seems on the surface to have a common shared meaning, but at a deeper level it appears profession specific.

This issue has gained much attention and reconsideration recently from various perspectives researching patient involvement, the empowerment of patients, patient safety, shared decision making, health literacy and/or constructing models of a health care team.

A seminal work, critically assessing the quality of citizen involvement by constructing a ladder of participation, was provided by Arnstein (1969). Eight stages were identified, ranging from very superficial and only apparent involvement to highly powerful participation in the decision-making processes. True citizen participation can only be acknowledged in the contexts of partnership relations, the redistribution of social power, and the enactment of citizen control. Focusing on patients as active consumers of health care services rather than supplicants, another influential consumerist model of exit, voice and loyalty, by Hirschman (1970), importantly demonstrated how organisations should work with their users if they are to remain successful. In addition to these classic models later versions included, e.g. Friedman and Miles' (2006) 12-step ladder model of engagement and Dent e.a. (2011) model of voice, choice and co-production, which were especially valuable in showing how "co-production only works effectively when there is mutual trust between user and professionals"; otherwise, such interactions might be dis-empowering and turn into proto-professionalization.

In 2001, Firth-Cozens, in the context of patient safety, wondered if patients themselves could ever be seen as team members. Howe (2006) addressed the same question, underscoring the importance of patient responsiveness. Becoming patient responsive may be associated with error prevention and a stronger organisational safety culture, increased motivation to change behaviour, enhanced adherence to advice, improved self-management, as well as increased patient satisfaction and likelihood of positive organisational changes. The patient clearly has to be actively involved.

It was found that active patient involvement strengthens clinical excellence. A patient-centred care improvement guide (Frampton e.a. 2008) states: "Patient-centred care is care organised around the patient. It is a model in which providers partner with patients and families to identify and satisfy the full range of patient needs and preferences [...] It does not replace excellent medicine – it both complements clinical excellence and contributes to it through effective partnerships and communication."

Reflecting Arnstein's emphasis on the redistribution of power, effective partnership also implies equal distribution of power within the decision-making process. Huby,

Brook, Thompson and Tierney (2007) determined that care routines or protocols in discharge planning can hinder active decision making. Schmitt (2011) recognized the important role of health workers' in supporting patients and their significant others in making informed choices. For some health situations with uncertain outcomes there may be a range of potential alternative clinical decisions which carry different kinds of risks. There is room for patient preferences within the shared decision-making process to find choices compatible with both patients' and professionals' values and preferences. Importantly, this is not only a matter of physician-patient interaction but also needs to be recognized in interprofessional contexts: patients should also be engaged, and their preferences acknowledged within interprofessional team decision making. There is a growing literature on patients' decision support (a systematic theory-based clinical strategy for helping people to engage in shared interprofessional decision making about their health care options) as well as patient decision aids (standardized, evidence-based tools that facilitate patients in understanding alternative choices, identifying their personal preferences, as well as forming and communicating their standpoints) (e.g. Legare 2011, Lown e.a. 2011, Col e.a. 2011).

Another prominent topic related to active patient participation is their (critical) health literacy. This notion comprises personal and social skills, determining the motivation and ability to gain access to, understand, and use information to promote and maintain good health (WHO 2009). Health literacy is a tool for patient empowerment; it facilitates social and political action and change, and aids in fighting inequalities in health care (Sykes, Wills, Rowlands & Popple 2013).

We have touched on some of the perspectives that have made space for lay people as active members of health care teams. There is a need to evolve the patient-centred care model to include users and/or their significant others as active members of health care teams. Focusing on social power relations within a health care team, Pahor (2014) developed three main models describing the historical development of health care teams: the Hierarchical/disease-centred model, the Patient-centred model, and the Health problem-centred model (see Figure 7).

We have mentioned some of the conceptual traps of the patient-centred model. It can imply a hierarchical relationship with patients at the centre of professional care but actually excluded from decision making, and only present as objects of treatment. In the health problem-centred model, social power is redistributed by shifting patients (their significant others and communities) to be alongside professionals, thus enabling shared decision making. It is important not to confuse this model with the traditional biomedical disease-centred perspective, precisely because it is patient-inclusive.

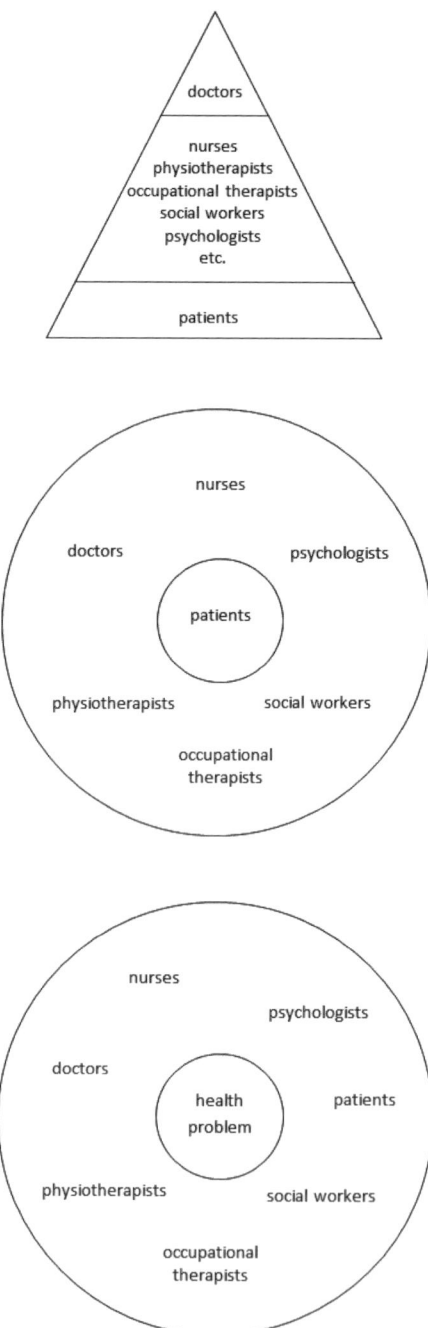

Figure 7: Three models of a health care team according to Pahor (2014): the Hierarchical disease-centred model (top), the Patient-centred model (middle), and the Health problem-centred model (bottom).

## Implications for education

As well as integrating the health problem-centred model into health professional education curricula, there are many other ways in lay people can actively participate in interprofessional courses. Lay people can be engaged as guests brought into the classroom to share experience, as experts by experience, expert informants, and as co-facilitators and educators. They can contribute to all stages of the process: planning, developing teaching resources, delivery and evaluation.

Towle and Godolphin (2013) reported on a project in which community (patient) educators delivered workshops themselves with faculty in a support role. The workshops were highly appreciated and valued. Patients have very specific expertise derived from their experience of illness, while faculty staff focus mainly on scientifically defined diseases. People living with chronic conditions are considered to be "experts by experience", but how can this expertise be integrated into educational practice? Community educators-patients educating others about what they consider to be important about their illness, without direct control of a faculty is a radical educational change. Students learn with rather than just about patients. This involves an important shift of perspective: community educators emphasize the need for care to be personalized, while in the classroom students are taught similarities rather than diversity. Barnes, Carpenter and Bailey (2006), in contrast, reported mixed reactions to healthcare users as trainers. Students found it very difficult to criticize their views and to challenge them; they were afraid to ask something wrong.

As already mentioned in discussion of shared decision making, there are particular skills to be learned and continually strengthened by professionals so as to be able to promote patients' involvement. This is especially significant for those patients who, do not want to be actively involved, perhaps because they do not have the confidence and skills. The 2012 Eurobarometer study on patient involvement (European Commission 2012) indicated that many patients saw the doctor as being someone beyond questioning, and they reported feeling uncomfortable giving feedback. In contrast, nurses were perceived as being much easier to communicate effectively with. Clearly, social power relations were strongly involved: nurses being perceived as much closer to patients, indicating much room for patient empowerment. An interprofessional team should be educated to be able to identify the most relevant options for the patient as well as to facilitate patient involvement in discussing and choosing among them. Legare (2011) identified the following components of patients' decision support: to provide the best information on the available options and their probable outcomes, to recognize patient's preferences, to acknowledge social and emotional influences that drive patient decisions, to consider patient's resources, and guide the patient through deliberations to make an informed and feasible choice.

The Faculty of Health Sciences of University of Ljubljana offers its students two courses that promote patient involvement. The elective inter-faculty course *Interprofessional Collaboration in a Health Care Team* (6 credits) started in 2011. Students of medicine, midwifery, nursing, occupational therapy, physiotherapy, psychology, radiography, sanitary engineering and social work participate in lectures, practice collaborative skills in small groups and work in teams to identify patients' problems and plan joint activities. In addition to the competences and areas of work of different professionals, they learn about theories of collaboration with a focus on the health problem-centred model of a health care team and special attention is paid to patient empowerment and involvement. In the first year the president of the Board of Patients at the University Medical Centre Ljubljana was invited as a guest lecturer to explain the first-hand experiences in promoting the user's voice. Student teams treated paper patients with specific multiple health issues. In 2013 interviews with live patients were introduced. Volunteers tell their stories and share their subjective experiences. At the end of the course, they are invited to hear and comment on the final reports of interprofessional student teams.

The elective course *Health Care Users' Perspective* (3 credits) was started in 2012. Through interviewing lay people, the aim of this course is to raise awareness and stimulate reflection concerning patients and users' lived experience of different health issues that students encounter from the professional academic viewpoint. The first year the course included students of sanitary engineering, nursing and occupational therapy. One group conducted interviews about the understanding and application of the patient's right to a second medical opinion. The other group contacted the Ljubljana Diabetes Association and had interviews with its members on the self-management of healthcare waste materials at home. As a follow-up to these interviews and at the Ljubljana Diabetes Association's initiative, a workshop with a group of its members was also carried out to promote good practice in health waste management among other members of the association. In 2013, students of sanitary engineering and nursing conducted interviews with their fellow students on smoking in front of the faculty building despite an explicit smoking ban. They reflected on the importance of understanding health promotion actions as well as on personal motivation and collective responsibility to observe the law. The other topic that year was lay people's perception and expectations of the students' own future professional field. They discovered different characteristics attributed to their future profession, found strength in positive images, discussed different strategies to surpass the negative stereotypes and became aware of the importance of the active involvement of lay people for the quality of their professional work.

## Does it matter what terms we use?

Throughout this text, thus far we have variously used the terms "patients", "users", "lay people", "experts", "professionals", etc. Are these just different words? Thomas (2010) argued that they are not neutral but imply social power. It led him to claim that by choosing one term over the other the speaker was engaged in an act of positioning, of allotting a person the place within the wider social context of social relations.

McLaughlin (2009) also claimed that terms and words construct identities, relationships, power dynamics and hierarchies of control. A "patient", for example, is by the very etymology of the word the one who waits, passively receives and accepts. The term "client" was described as the user of services, also passive and dependent on professionals but attributed more choice than a patient. The term "customer or consumer" reflects the commercialization of health care, where health and care are commodities being bought and/or sold. It implies even more freedom and choice for the customer. The positive aspect of the term "service user" is its strong association with participation. An "expert by experience" is a term underscoring the importance of living with a certain health condition and well as the special kind of knowledge that is generated from it. Professionals work on the basis of objective data, but patients know themselves best, contribute their subjective feelings and experiences. The meanings of the words used need to be considered carefully. Terms may gain new connotations in different contexts of use and in time. They need to be constantly critically reflected upon. One way to avoid expert imposition is to ask the persons (or groups of people) themselves how they wish to be referred to.

We have also touched upon the different interpretations of the concept patient-centred care, showing how it has been analysed as patient inclusive or expert patronizing. Finally, our deliberation also needs to be focused on the term inter-professional (education, practice or team).

## Redefinition of interprofessionalism?

As we have seen from the student answers at the beginning of this text, the term "interprofessional" can be misleading in a way that excludes lay people from active collaborative care. In another study, we also considered some lay people's viewpoints on collaboration in health care (Kavčič, Pahor & Domajnko 2015). Comparing the proto-professional student voice with the lay one, a contradiction in perceptions emerged quite clearly. A patronizing professional attitude towards patients predominated in students' answers, while there was a strong stress on partnership and active involvement of both sides in people's views. Despite quite widespread unclear and poor understanding of patient involvement (i.e. equating it with medical compliance and patients providing only basic information and less widely to include interactive dialogue), the Eurobarometer study (European Commission 2012) also identified public voices wanting more balanced relationships in healthcare. This need was most evident for the chronically ill (who already have more experiences in self-monitoring), younger patients and those with better education, who had higher expectations of their own involvement in decision making. Gordon, Feldman and Leonard (2014) convey stories reflecting experiences in which highly educated patients, and even health care experts found it difficult to ask questions or advocate for themselves or their important ones due to a fear of being labelled "difficult". The positive impact on the clinical outcomes when patients were listened to is also reported. The only way to include patients in the team is to let their voice be at the centre of the conversation.

There are multiple ways of explaining the persistence of patronizing (proto)expert attitudes towards patients. From the historical-cultural viewpoint, the traditional hierarchical patterns of social relations are still powerfully framing health care practice. They also influence student professional socialization during their clinical practice. However and more relevant to this text, sometimes there is also the lack of clarity and congruity in definitions of interprofessional collaboration that students encounter during the academic educational process.

In literature reviews on patient-centredness or interprofessionalism, it was detected that active patient involvement was frequently only presupposed and left undefined and ambiguous. If not expressed explicitly, it may help perpetuate patronizing interpretations of professionals collaborating to provide (in their opinion) the best care for the patients. In the conceptualization of patients as experts by experience (partners to experts by profession), it became clear that we are all health workers, but lay people, their significant others and sometimes whole communities are in a weaker position to establish their place within health care teams. They need empowerment and explicit support to actively participate.

Patients and their significant others as actively involved partners in the health care team seem to be among goals, values and visions of the promoters of interprofessional collaboration. Since this is not self-evident, it requires a straightforward approach and a clear statement. For example, Herbert (2005) wrote: "Collaborative patient-centred practice is a practice orientation, a way of health care professionals working together and with patients. It involves the continuous interaction of two or more professionals or disciplines, organised into a common effort, to solve or explore common issues with the best possible participation of the patient." The WHO Framework for action on interprofessional education and collaborative practice (WHO 2010), as well as networks such as EIPEN and CAIPE (Centre for the Advancement of Interprofessional Education) promote interprofessional learning that actively involves service users and local communities as essential partners.

In clinical practice, educational activities and research, we constantly need to reflect on the terminology we use. It reveals our deeper presupposed conceptualizations and values. When talking about interprofessional teams, who exactly is included? When do the patient or/and their important others or even communities join in? How do all team members relate in terms of social power? In this text, we have attempted to explain that the term "interprofessional" may stand in strong opposition to non-professionals. At the heart of the idea of collaboration, there seems to be the notion of seamless practice stemming from good collaboration of all the stakeholders, non-professionals included, on equal social grounds. Maintaining emphasis on the notion of collaboration among different health-related professions, it seems that the term "interprofessional collaboration" needs to be modified strongly by being performed together with rather than for people, in other words, by being refered to as "lay people (and their significant others and communities) empowering and inclusive interprofessional collaboration".

# Literature

Arnstein SR (1969). A ladder of citizen participation. *Journal of the American Institute of Planners, 35*, 216-224.

Barnes D, Carpenter J & Bailey D (2006). Partnerships with service users in interprofessional education for community mental health: a case study. *Journal of Interprofessional Care, 14*, 189-200.

Col N, Bozzuto L, Kirkegaard P, Koelewijn-van Loon M, Majeed H, Ng CJ & Pacheco-Huergo V (2011). Interprofessional education about shared decision making for patients in primary care settings. *Journal of Interprofessional Care, 25*, 409-415.

Dent M, Fallon C, Wendt C, Vuori J, Pahor M, de Pietro C & Silva S (2011). Medicine and user involvement within European healthcare: A typology for European comparative research, *The International Journal of Clinical Practice, 65*, 1218-1220.

European Commission (2012). Patient involvement: Eurobarometer qualitative study (2012). Retrieved from http://ec.europa.eu/public_opinion/archives/quali/ql_5937_patient_en.pdf

Firth-Cozens J (2001). Cultures for improving patient safety through learning: The role of teamwork. *Quality in Health Care, 10* (Suppl II), ii26-ii31.

Frampton S, Guastello S, Brady C, Hale M, Horowitz S, Bennett Smith S & Stone S (2008). *Patient-centered care improvement guide*. Derby, Connecticut: Planetree.

Friedman A & Miles S (2006). *Stakeholders: Theory and practice*. Oxford University Press.

Gachoud D, Albert M, Kuper A, Stroud L & Reeves S (2012). Meanings and perceptions of patient-centeredness in social work, nursing and medicine: A comparative study. *Journal of Interprofessional Care, 26*, 484-490.

Gordon S, Feldman DL & Leonard M (2014). *Collaborative caring: Stories and reflections on teamwork in health care*. New York: Cornell University Press.

Herbert CP (2005). Changing the culture: Interprofessional education for collaborative patient-centred practice in Canada. *Journal of Interprofessional Care,* , Suppl 1, 1-4.

Hirschman AO (1970). *Exit, voice, and loyalty: Responses to decline in firms, organizations, and states*. Harvard University Press.

Howe A (2006). Can the patient be on our team? An operational approach to patient involvement in interprofessional approaches to safe care. *Journal of Interprofessional Care, 20*, 527-534.

Huby G, Brook JH, Thompson A & Tierney A (2007). Capturing the concealed: Interprofessional practice and older patients' participation in decision-making about discharge after acute hospitalization. *Journal of Interprofessional Care, 21*, 55-67.

Kavčič M, Pahor M & Domajnko B (2015). User involvement in Slovenian healthcare. *Journal of Health Organization and Management* – in press.

Legare F (2011). Interprofessional education for interprofessional practice about patients' decision support/patients' decision aids. *Journal of Interprofessional Care, 25*, 399-400.

Lown BA, Kryworuchko J, Bieber C, Lillie DM, Kelly C, Berger B & Loh A (2011). Continuing professional development for interprofessional teams supporting patients in healthcare decision making. *Journal of Interprofessional Care, 25*, 401-408.

McLaughlin H (2009). What's in a Name: 'Client', 'Patient', 'Customer', 'Consumer', 'Expert by experience', 'Service User' – What's Next? *British Journal of Social Work, 39*, 1101-1117.

Pahor M (Ed.) (2014). *Zavezniki za zdravje: medpoklico sodelovanje v zdravstvenih timih [Partners for health: Interprofessional collaboration in health care teams]*. Ljubljana: UL-ZF.

Schmitt MH (2011). Supporting patients' decision making: Interprofessional perspectives. *Journal of Interprofessional Care, 25*, 397-398.

Sykes S, Wills J, Rowlands G & Popple K (2013). Understanding critical health literacy: A concept analysis. *BMC Public Health, 13*, 150.

Thomas J (2010). Service users, carers and issues for collaborative practice. In KC Pollard, J Thomas & M Miers (Eds.). *Understanding interprofessional working in health and social care* (171-186). London: Palgrave-Macmillan.

Towle A & Godolphin W (2013). Patients as educators: Interprofessional learning for patient-centred care. *Medical Teacher, 35*, 219-225.

WHO (2009). Health Literacy and Health Promotion. Retrieved from http://www.who.int/healthpromotion/conferences/7gchp/Track1_Inner.pdf

WHO (2010). Framework for Action on Interprofessional Education & Collaborative Practice. Retrieved from http://www.who.int/hrh/nursing_midwifery/en/

# Creating spaces for interprofessional learning: Strategic revision of a common IPL curriculum in undergraduate programmes

Annika Lindh Falk, Johanna Dahlberg, Mattias Ekstedt, Annika Heslyk, Per Whiss and Madeleine Abrandt Dahlgren

## Responding to changing conditions

The Faculty of Medicine and Health Sciences at Linköping University has a long tradition of interprofessional learning activities for students in all undergraduate programmes. As a response to new global challenges including the changing health care system, and to institutional challenges in the shift to a new generation of teachers, and increasing numbers of undergraduate students, a group of professional educators across the faculty was assigned to re-think and revise the existing interprofessional curriculum for all undergraduate programmes, i.e. Biomedical Laboratory Science, Medical Biology, Medicine, Nursing, Occupational Therapy, Physiotherapy, and Speech and Language Pathology. The focus of this chapter is to explore the change strategy and process of developing the new curriculum. We also provide a description of the structure and a summary of the content in the renewed curriculum.

## The structure of the developmental process

The task force structured the work process according to a theoretical model for interprofessional curriculum development as described by Lee e.a. (2013, Figure 8). This model emphasizes the importance of considering four interrelated dimensions in the process of developing a new curriculum. These dimensions are i) future orientation of health practices, ii) knowledge, competencies, capabilities and practices, iii) teaching, learning and assessment approaches and practices, and iv) institutional delivery. The task force started with an analysis of the first dimension of the model of interprofessional curriculum development. This dimension addresses the 'why' question of educational planning and concerns the necessity to connect the curriculum to the world of practice and the changing demands in the workplace of all health sectors.

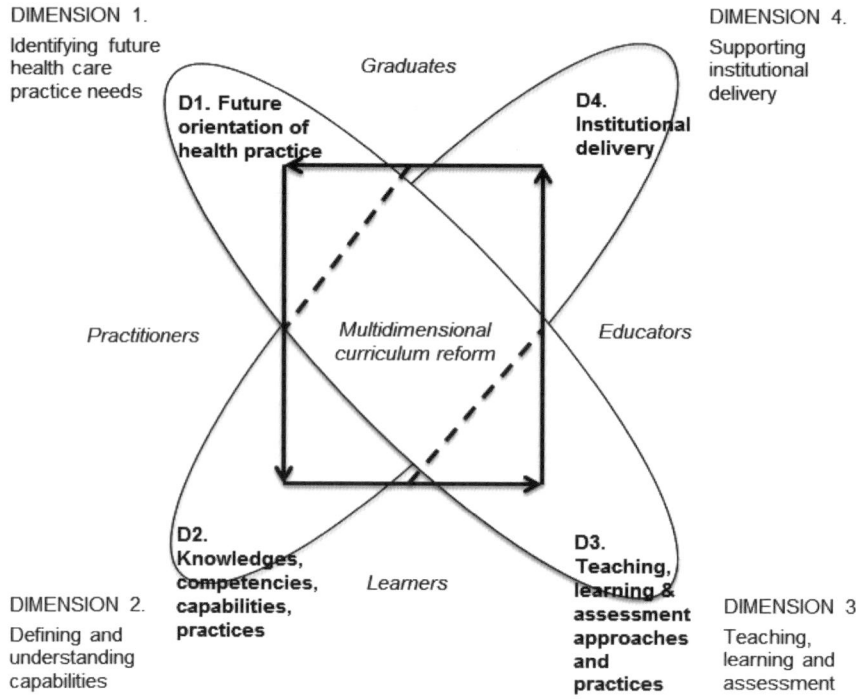

Figure 8. Model for interprofessional curriculum development (Lee e.a. 2013).

Against the backdrop of changing conditions for health care, there is a global call for strategic changes in professional programmes in medicine and health. The Lancet Commission report (Frenk e.a. 2010) lists a number of aspects that affect the conditions for sustainable health care globally. These global issues are: how to secure sustainable use of financial and personal resources, how to establish partnership models of healthcare delivery, how to improve patient safety, and how to establish effective teamwork and collaborative practice, all of which are part of the agenda for educational developers. Other issues are gaps and inequalities in health care within and between countries, emerging infectious diseases, environmental and behavioural risk factors, the rapid demographic shift towards an aging population, and thus, an aging workforce in the healthcare system. Professional health care programmes need to be adapted to meet these challenges in order to improve collaboration and security in health care.

The Lancet commission argues that there is a need for a new professionalism and a new set of skills-based criteria to classify the competence of health professionals. Competency-based curricula and interprofessional education have also been promoted globally by policy makers as a necessity to meet the demands of future health professionals (World Health Organisation 2010). While the shift to competency-based learning outcomes through the Bologna process is well known for professional educators across Europe, interprofessional education (IPE) is still often not given specific attention in many programmes for education of health professionals (Frenk e.a. 2010). Interprofessional education has been defined as curricular activities in which students from different professional programmes learn from, with and about each other (CAIPE 1997, Thistletwaite 2012).

Reflection on the local state-of-the-art of teaching and learning at the Faculty of Medicine and Health Sciences at Linköping University, Sweden, provided a starting point for analysis of aspects that resonate with the global needs of promoting collaboration and safety in health care education for the future, and aspects that needed to be developed and changed. A problem-based approach to learning and an interprofessional curriculum are the cornerstones of a common pedagogic approach, encompassing all programmes since the start 1986 (Hammar, Bergdahl & Öhman 2006). The common approach has brought about a student- and learning-centred discourse within the faculty. In accordance with the focus on learning, we will use the term interprofessional learning throughout the chapter for all educational activities described. The pedagogy emphasises integration in several dimensions by organisation of recurrent interprofessional learning activities over time, which could be seen as an established basic principle that enables collaboration between students during their undergraduate studies. Further, integration of the content of study is accomplished through a problem-based and thematic organisation of the subject matter as well as the integration of theoretical and clinical parts of the education through recurrent clinical placements in various health care contexts. These features of the pedagogical approach resonate with the Lancet commission recommendation of competency-based and interprofessional curricula. The applied approach to education has proved to be successful over the years, acknowledged by evaluations through the Swedish Higher Education Authority. Hence, our starting point for re-thinking the organisation of the interprofessional curriculum is sustainable educational practice where all students are involved in recurrent learning activities throughout their study programmes. In short, the prevailing curriculum comprises three mandatory modules of activities:

- A common start in interprofessional study (7 weeks) to establish a common ground for professional work within health care,
- A clinically situated quality improvement scenario (2 weeks) at the intermediate level of the programmes,
- A clinical placement at a student led interprofessional training ward (IPTW) (2 weeks) at the final stage of the programmes.

The present organisation with seven consecutive weeks of interprofessional study prior to the start of programme specific learning activities has been subject to much debate. The internal discussion within the faculty, as conveyed in colloquia and through evaluations from students and teachers over the years, have repeatedly pointed to the need of clarifying the objectives of the IPL activities and the relationship to the programme specific studies. The separation of interprofessional learning activities from professional learning activities seems to make it difficult for students at the initial level of the programmes to see the relevance of the interprofessional studies. Such experiences have also been confirmed in research on interprofessional learning, following a similar curriculum model (see Ekeli 2013, Reeves, Tassone, Parker, Wagner & Simmons 2012).

The present problem-based approach to learning has also been debated in the faculty. One effect, among others, of the ongoing generation shift of teachers in the faculty is that many of the champions and founding fathers of the original idea from the outset are gone or not active anymore (Areskog 2009). The need of revitalisation of the pedagogical idea behind the working forms in the faculty has become obvious. Another aspect that brings consequences for pedagogical approach and working forms is the increasing student numbers, comprising an intake of 450 students each semester are three times as many today than at the launch in 1986. The numbers of faculty members have not increased at corresponding pace, which makes the teaching load larger for each individual teacher. In total, the number of teachers in the faculty is about 300. The large numbers of students make the complexity of logistics and material arrangements of interprofessional study an administrative challenge of considerable amount.

The result of the analysis of the first dimension of the model for interprofessional curriculum development lead us to be assured that in terms of social and material arrangements for interprofessional learning the foundation in place constitutes a robust and sustainable ground as a starting point for change. Important areas in need of development were identified in how to accomplish

- clearer learning objectives for interprofessional competence to enhance awareness of their relevance and
- tighter integration of interprofessional and programme specific elements.

The next phase of the task force work was to analyse the second dimension of the curriculum model concerning the 'what' question - what should be the content of the intended learning outcomes for interprofessional competence. What knowledge, capabilities and attributes are required of health care professionals? It is important here to take into account the relational nature of competence - changes in health care services brings about changes in practices, identities and expertise of professionals (Lee e.a. 2013).

These changes also bring consequences for what should be included in the curriculum and part of the education of health care professionals for the future. The task force located existing intended IPL outcomes in course outlines for all undergraduate programmes on the local university level, as well as on the national level. In addition, intended learning outcomes were also defined based on the IPEC (2011) competency-based framework for interprofessional practice, with four competency domains: Values/Ethics, Roles/Responsibilities, Interprofessional communication, and Teams/Teamwork. We also identified a fifth domain of competence: Pedagogy and Learning. Competence in pedagogy and learning may enhance the professionals' articulating and understanding how and what the team learns "with, from and about" each other in collaboration, and for understanding patients' perspectives and their learning needs. Competence in pedagogy and learning may also provide the necessary awareness and the tools needed to involve patients/clients in decisions about their own care.

We elaborated and developed the framework to construct an interprofessional curriculum that would fit with the educational objectives for the professional health care programmes at the Faculty of Medicine and Health Sciences in Linköping. In order to work as a framework in an educational setting, competency-based learning objectives were formulated with progression over the course of the curriculum for each competency domain. As a result of the Bologna process and the process of higher education harmonisation in Europe, the intended learning outcomes of education should express the desired knowledge and understanding, competence and skills, judgement and approach that the students are expected to achieve. This meant that learning objectives were formulated for interprofessional activities on the initial, intermediate and final level of the undergraduate programmes, for all identified IPEC competency domains. In addition to creating increasing complexity of learning tasks, we also increased complexity through exposing students to various contexts in which the competences should be enacted. One example pertaining to the domain of *Roles and responsibilities* is that students at the initial level of IPL are expected to learn to identify roles and responsibilities in their own tutorial group. At the final level, competences regarding roles and responsibilities are expected to be demonstrated in the clinical setting, comprising the roles and responsibilities in a patient-centred approach. Finally, the framework was completed through the addition of a portfolio system for assessment of interprofessional competence, as we describe in the following paragraphs.

In the following section we move on to the analysis of the third dimension of the curriculum development, representing the 'how' question, i.e. appropriate teaching, learning and assessment strategies for interprofessional learning. Also in this dimension, we started out by a review of the literature on which pedagogical approach is best suited to achieve interprofessional learning.

Reeves and co-workers (2012) point out, in an overview of research on IPE, the need for an interactive approach to learning to achieve interprofessional skills. Barr, Koppel, Reeves, Hammick and Freeth (2012) described the various interactive approaches often used in IPE contexts. These are referred to as 'exchange based', i.e. approaches that emphasize dialogue, including seminars; 'observation based', i.e. joint study of patients/clients; 'action-based', which is defined as problem-based learning; 'simulation based', which involves simulated clinical practice; 'practice based learning,' such as interprofessional clinical practice; as well as e-learning, such as web-based discussions. Reeves and colleagues emphasise that the selection of an interactive educational approach to IPL depends on the objectives, participants and the resources available. Combining several approaches can lead to a learning environment that is more motivating and stimulating for students (Reeves e.a. 2012, Wilhelmsson 2011).

An analysis of the knowledge base of PBL as a teaching approach for IPL shows that PBL rests on several scientific and theoretical approaches that can be described as a growing realization over time of how student learning can be improved. There are also strong influences from cognitive theories and psychological research on the functioning of human memory and its consequences for learning (e.g. Norman & Schmidt 1992, Schraw 1998). Phenomenographic research on learning in higher education (e.g. Marton, Hounsell & Entwistle 1984) has been important to understand how PBL as an educational design can support deep oriented approaches to learning. The pragmatic, cognitive and phenomenographic perspectives have also been supplemented with a social constructivist perspective that emphasizes the social dimension of learning, in which meaning is constructed in interaction with others (Savery & Duffy 1995).

The predominant research-based and theoretically based rationale for PBL as an applied pedagogical approach has focused on students' thinking and learning processes, and what can be done in terms of pedagogical arrangements in order to support learning. Recent research emphasizes that the one-sided focus on cognitive processes is not sufficient for designing modern professional programmes to meet future requirements. It is also necessary to understand how the social and material arrangements influence and make learning possible (Fenwick 2010). Dahlgren (2009) describes the most important features and principles of PBL as:

- Ownership of the learning task, i.e. the students' own questions and autonomous learning drive the learning.
- Contextualisation of key concepts, namely the theoretical concepts is studied in a meaningful, real-life context.
- Interactive learning environment, i.e. students develops knowledge in dialogue with one another and with tutors.

- Learning as a content in itself to increase and support students' awareness of their own learning, i.e. reflection and metacognition is emphasized.

In our audit of the interprofessional curriculum activities already in place, we consider it is important to maintain the structure of learning in small tutorial groups, where students are responsible for, and direct their learning, based on their own stated learning objectives. Such a structure contributes to a depth-oriented approach to learning and maintains and improves motivation for learning among students. Previous research has shown that if students lack opportunities to influence the content of their studies, a surface approach to learning is more likely to appear among students, which is less favourable to learning (Marton e.a. 1998).

In modern research on human learning, there is a growing understanding that learning is a contextual process in which the contextual features also largely determine how people learn (Lave & Wenger 1991, Säljö 2000). In PBL, real-life scenarios are used as a basis for learning. The reason for this is to encourage the students to identify their existing knowledge as well as their learning needs, and to create a meaningful context related to the student's future career. The basic idea is not only to learn about the context and applications, but also to learn by experiencing the context (Dahlgren 2009). By starting the process of inter-professional learning through scenarios, the students learn to identify relevant aspects that are important for their professional and interprofessional perspective and understanding. Against the background of educational research and theories of learning it is reasonable to assume that to deepen students understanding presenting theoretical concepts distinguished by their relevance in their common context, is a better strategy than lecture-based training design where the relevance of the theoretical concepts can be difficult to discern for the student.

An even distribution of different professions avoids any dominance conditions (Reeves e.a. 2012). Keeping groups together over time is beneficial for the development of interaction in the group. IPL groups held over a shorter time with more frequent membership changes place greater demands on the supervisor's competence. Reeves and colleagues (2012) have also summarized the requirements for tutorial skills for IPL as reported in the literature. IPL tutors should have experience of interprofessional collaboration, a deep understanding of interactive learning methods, knowledge of group dynamics, an enthusiasm for interprofessional learning and collaboration, the confidence to work in interprofessional teams, act as a role model, able to reflect the collaborative learning, and be flexible in relation to different groups.

Learning is supported by the tutor's attitude, questions and interventions aimed to challenge students to critically examine their own knowledge, their sources, their cooperation in formulating goals for their learning, and in discussing their newfound knowledge. Challenging students to critically assess their performance is seen as a way to make the learning process accessible to reflection so that students can develop and improve their capacity for learning. The indisputable importance of reflecting on their own thinking and action has been clearly pointed out by several authors (e.g. Schön 1987, Schraw 1998). Dahlgren (2009) suggests that learning can also be described as a social process, where members of a community of learning discuss and clarify the meaning of phenomena and problems in their practice. In this respect, reflection individually or in groups over a just finished learning task is seen as a process similar to what happens in a group in health care when evaluating what it has accomplished, for example, during a working day.

To sum up, PBL to achieve interprofessional competencies appear in the light of the literature review as a fruitful pedagogical approach (Dahlgren 2009, Reeves e.a. 2012). It is important in the practical arrangements that both formal and informal learning situations are designed to facilitate mutual interaction between the members of the group, whether it be professional or interprofessional learning. One conclusion we draw is that it is important for faculty teachers to develop skills and support so that they can vary their teaching within the framework of problem-based learning.

After a review of the literature, our conclusion was that PBL remains a robust and suitable approach to integrate IPL in the professional programmes at the Faculty of Medicine and Health Sciences. Although there is no clear evidence for the best time to introduce IPL we argue that it is important to start early so that students can be socialised into a shared knowledge base about the health care system, a shared set of values, and the role and function of the various professions within this system as a common ground for their further studies.

Further, we are implementing the use of an individual IPL-portfolio as the form of assessment aiming at enhancing integration of interprofessional and professional learning. Portfolio is a well-established form of assessment, which in recent years has been commonly used in healthcare education. The assessment form builds on students' documentation and gathering of evidence for their learning during a course, together with their personal reflections on their learning experiences. The portfolio can be purely formative, mainly aiming at supporting student learning, and/or it may also have a summative function, which is used as the assessment of a specific part of the course, as we propose here.

The pedagogical rationale for the use of portfolios as an assessment strategy is that professional competence includes capability to critically assess one's own performance as a basis for improvement and development in a lifelong learning perspective (Boud & Falchikov 2006). In this way, the assessment form can be said to be constructively aligned (Biggs & Tang 2011) with learning objectives involving the development of a critical approach. Studies also show that students' estimation of their own performance usually corresponds well with the teacher's, and it is possible for the student to calibrate the ability to estimate the performance over time (Boud, Thompson & Lawson 2013). A systematic literature review on the use of the portfolio as a tool for learning and assessment (Buckley e.a. 2009) shows that the use of the portfolio positively impacts on student learning and understanding, self-awareness and reflectivity. In this way, the assessment form in itself drives the development and learning (O'Sullivan e.a. 2012). This applies especially if the students are involved from the start of their training and if the portfolio is linked to the learning objectives.

The next phase of our process was an analysis of the fourth dimension of the curriculum development model, i.e. how to support institutional delivery, and how to integrate the local university structure and culture in the shaping of curriculum design and delivery. The model for curriculum development (Lee e.a. 2013) emphasizes the importance of paying attention to the views of different stakeholders in the process, i.e. teachers, students, practitioners and graduates. A review of the literature on barriers and enablers for IPL supports the idea of mutual involvement as key factors of success on the governmental, institutional and individual level (Lawlis e.a. 2014). Enablers at the governmental level are the establishment of collaborative groups from different higher education institutions and organisations, stakeholder commitment, shared ownership and unified goals and government funding. The governmental level in our case basically consisted of learning objectives concerning interprofessional collaboration being emphasised in all national programme outlines for professional health care education in Sweden. In addition, in their quality assessment of medical programmes in Sweden 2014 the Swedish Higher Education Authority focused on interprofessional collaborative skills. The result of the evaluation was that three out of six programmes did not pass due to lack of learning arrangements for interprofessional collaboration. At the institutional level, Lawlis, Anson and Greenfield (2014) show that enablers of IPL are a) funding of institutions, b) organisational structures within higher education institutions developed, and c) the existence of faculty development programmes. In our case, funding was already available through the existing interprofessional curriculum, and accordingly also organisational structures in place. However, to address the generation shift in the faculty, further faculty development focusing on PBL and IPL tutoring is needed. Adjustments of available faculty development courses are being done, and new courses are being planned and subsequently implemented. Enablers of IPL on the individual level identified by Lawlis e.a. (2014) are skills and enthusiasm of the staff, role models and champions, a shared understanding and vision for interprofessional education, commitment, and showing of equal status regardless of position and background. We can identify with all of these enablers as part of the background and history of successful implementation of an IPL curriculum in Linköping, and it is important to maintain and foster this spirit in the ongoing generation shift of the faculty. We also emphasise the importance of bringing the students on board, sharing the learning vision of the faculty.

So far, we have described how we analysed the content and structure of the existing IPL curriculum. In the following, we will also account for the process of involving different stakeholders in the process of rethinking and revising the curriculum. As part of a strategy for developing pedagogical awareness of the task force, a series of three seminars were given by international educational experts visiting the faculty. The seminars were open to all teachers in the faculty and the visiting experts also acted as critical friends. The seminars concerned learning and assessment in higher education in particular and perspectives on professional learning more generally. During the year of development of the new curriculum, the Deans of the Faculty have been in close dialogue with the task force, and the work in progress has also continuously been presented in different forums to involve all stakeholders in the process. Some of these forums are the board for undergraduate education, the monthly faculty colloquium, the faculty board, and the student union. To involve all stakeholders in the process and decision, the final proposal for the new interprofessional curriculum was sent out on referral. The responses to the proposal were collated and discussed and the viewpoints from the stakeholders were incorporated in the Faculty board's final decision about a revised curriculum. As a next step in the process, a group of representatives for each programme, the student union and the local health care provider was assigned to implement the new curriculum.

## The new curriculum of IPL

In the new interprofessional curriculum we have focused on the five competency domains as both learning goals and course contents. Students will acquire interprofessional knowledge, skills and abilities by taking part in interprofessional learning activities and through the critical examination of the theoretical foundations and empirical evidence of the needs for interprofessional collaboration in health care. We suggest that the interprofessional identification process should start parallel to the professional identification. The new IPL-curriculum comprises of three modules; I) "Professionalism in Health Care" during the initial level of the programmes (4 weeks), II) "Quality Improvement in Healthcare Practice" at the intermediate level (2 weeks), and III) "Professional Perspectives in Collaboration" (2 weeks) at the final level of the programmes.

The first module of our IPL-curriculum - *Professionalism in Healthcare* - starts week seven during the first semester in all programmes. The first and last week are organised as fulltime studies with four weeks in between organised as halftime. Therefore, module 1 will stretch over six weeks in total to allow the students more time to reflect upon their interprofessional experience. In addition, each programme will run programme specific courses which will be related to and integrated with the IPL curriculum. The aim of this enhanced integration is to underline that IPL competences are an integrated part of each profession.

Following our PBL based curriculum approach, students work in small (7-9 students) tutorial groups, with realistic web-based and multimedia enhanced scenarios (EDIT) as starting points for their learning. The groups are guided by trained tutors (Persson, Fyrenius & Bergdahl 2010). All programmes start each week with a shared scenario designed to trigger questions relevant for both programme specific purposes as well as for the interprofessional purposes. The programme specific tutorial groups are followed by interprofessional tutorial groups, where questions relevant for IPL will be discussed. We suggest that engaging the same tutors in the IPL activity as in the programme specific activity will enforce connection between interprofessional and professional learning. The scenarios are designed to stimulate learning within the five competency domains on which the IPL curriculum rests. In addition to tutorial group sessions and self-directed learning, the students also engage in lectures, seminars, communication skills exercise as well as contact with patients focusing on the role of the different professions.

The second module, *Quality Improvement in Health Care Practice*, is placed at the intermediate level of the interprofessional curricula. As we mentioned earlier, health care professionals should have competencies in improvement of quality and safety (IQS) to achieve better patient outcome in health care practice (Frenk e.a. 2010) and we argue it is important for students to achieve these competencies during their education. The module is situated at the end of the final year, engaging at least 4 professional programmes depending on autumn and spring semester period. This module is organised in close collaboration with the regional health care provider to ensure realistic scenarios for the students to work with and to recognize that learning is an integral part of everyday working practice.

The intended learning outcomes for the second module have two different foci. Firstly, the students are required to apply methods and tools from models of IQS and analyse the complexity in quality improvement processes. Secondly, the students expected to reflect upon their own professional knowledge in relation to others in order to describe and discern interprofessional competences and also discuss how interprofessional collaboration can affect the quality and safety in health care.

During a period of two weeks the students come together in interprofessional tutorial groups of 7-9 students. Key persons from different clinical settings such as health care centres, laboratory units and clinical wards are engaged in the process of identifying and selecting appropriate projects, originating in everyday clinical practices. Each group of students are presented with a unique clinical scenario. Examples of scenarios that have been subject to quality improvement work by student teams are how to develop better routines at the ward rounds; how to increase accessibility for patients to acute care settings and how to improve hygiene routines. The students discuss and clarify the specific focus of the problem, what to measure, how to perform the measurements, what kind of data that could be of interest, and suggested interventions. The Plan-Do-Study-Act-cycle (PDSA) is one of several important tools for IQS being used. Tutorial group meetings, a clinical visit for data collection and an inquiry seminar, where the students critically discussed their issues together with students from other groups, are organised during the two weeks. Finally, suggested improvements are presented in a final written assignment and an oral presentation at the specific clinic. During the module, students are supervised by an academic tutor and the key person from the clinic.

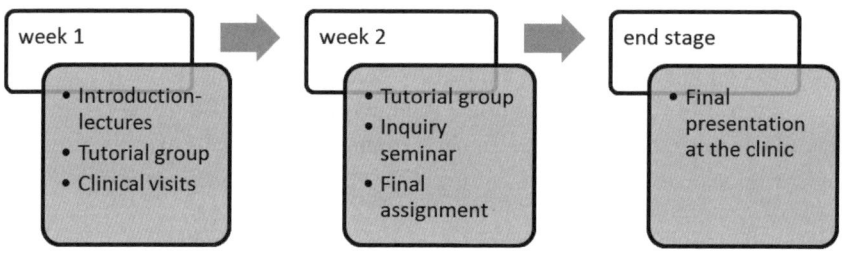

Figure 9: Structure of the IPL module on quality improvement in health care practice.

The third module of the IPL curriculum, *Professional Perspectives in Collaboration*, is placed at the final level of the programmes. This module comprises 2 weeks of fulltime study and is mandatory for five programmes. Interprofessional training wards (IPTW) were introduced in 1996 as a means for practising and learning teamwork and communication. The perceived value of the placement persists in recurrent student evaluations; hence, the task force was determined to maintain the concept of students learning and practice teamwork in a clinical placement as a fruitful way of providing for interprofessional learning. A group of students are scheduled to act as specific health care teams at an orthopaedic or geriatric hospital ward, covering daytime and evening shifts. At the IPTW, all students are responsible for all aspects of care such as making beds, and helping patients with personal hygiene, as well as for their own professional tasks. The number of occupational therapy and physiotherapy students is lower than the number of students from the medicine and nursing programmes, which means that these students work across the teams in the ward, being responsible for rehabilitation issues for all patients, irrespectively of team. Learning goals at the IPTW integrate knowledge, skills and attitudes from all the competency domains, meaning that the student teams organise and manage the medical issues, the daily care and the rehabilitation. In that sense, the IPTW is a means of practising common sets of values for patient-centred care as much as practising collaboration and specific professional tasks. Research (Lindh

Falk, Hult, Hammar, Hopwood & Abrandt Dahlgren 2013) shows that the proximity between the students appeared to break down the professional silos and strengthened the relationships between the student groups in collaboration with the patient.

From previous experiences and repeated evaluations by students, we know that the two week placement seems to enable students to reach the intended learning outcomes, even though students have frequently said that a third week would be provide the full experience of a functioning health care team. This is probably perfectly reasonable, taking into account the time needed for the team to get established during the first week of the placement. Due to the logistical complexity, there is currently no possibility of prolonging the placement with a third week. Against the backdrop of the changing conditions for future health care, hospital care will not be the dominating form in the health care system; alternative forms will be used more frequently, such as primary health care centres, home care settings, and community-based care. In the transformation of professional health care education, it is important that these alternative forms of care also reflected in the educational setting.

## Assessment

The aim of the IPL portfolio is that the students should become aware of and demonstrate that they have attained the skills and abilities that are stated as IPL learning objectives. The content should reflect evidence of the students' knowledge and skills, both theoretical and practical. The portfolio is designed so that it both allows assessment of each sequence of IPL activities, and acts as a device for meaningful integration of interprofessional learning over time across the different IPL activities. At the outset of each IPL activity, the students will reflect on the fundamental learning objectives of IPL in relation to the programme-specific learning activities. This reflection will be documented and make up the foundation for the IPL portfolio. The students are also recommended to discuss with their tutors about what to include as evidence of learning in the portfolio.

A student-centred learning approach also includes the student as involved in assessing their own learning processes. After completion of each IPL activity, the student should formulate their learning and progression in a number of distinct points and make a summary description of the portfolio content in this respect. For formative support of the students' personal development the portfolio also includes a section that is personal and is not subject to assessment. In order for the assessment to be reliable, it requires that the various examiners are familiar with how the portfolio task has been formulated and what should be valued in the portfolio. The examiners also need to have the relevant knowledge of how the content should be assessed. The portfolio assessment has to be perceived as fair and safe for both students and teachers and there should be clear instructions developed for how the portfolio should be documented and assessed.

## Concluding reflections

The re-thinking of the interprofessional curriculum can be summarised in six points:

- Articulation of a common curriculum based on a competency framework for IPL
- Common progressive intended interprofessional learning outcomes for each competency domain
- Enhanced integration of interprofessional and professional learning elements
- Introducing a competency domain of pedagogy and learning
- Establishing new sites for clinical interprofessional collaboration
- The development of a common portfolio assessment for interprofessional learning.

From more than 25 years of experience of interprofessional education at the Faculty of Medicine and Health sciences, we know from student and teacher evaluations, that a common assumption is that interprofessional activities takes time from the professional learning. Faresjö, Wilhelmsson, Pelling, Dahlgen and Hammar (2007), however, showed in a national survey of the medical programmes in Sweden, that the interprofessional learning did not jeopardise medical skills of our students. Östergren, Kaviani, Thorvaldsen, Krook-Brandt and Dahlgren (2009) confirmed these results in a comparison of national internship test results. In our revision, the intention has been to emphasise interprofessional learning as an integrated part of the professional programmes. Hence, the assessment of interprofessional competence will not be assessed separately, but integrated with the assessment of the professional learning.

In our revision work, we added a fifth domain of competence for interprofessional collaboration, aspiring to stimulate patient-centred care. Provision of patient-centred care is at the heart and the goal of interprofessional teamwork, and the nature of the relationship between the patient and the team of health professionals is seen as central to competency development for interprofessional collaborative practice. A very reasonable question to ask is then how the discourse of interprofessional collaboration intersects with the discourse of person-centred or patient-centred care. In a recent article published earlier this year, Fox and Reeves (2015) suggest that the discourse of patient-centred work and interprofessional collaboration does not take into account the conditions under which health professionals work – the inequities in social, economic and political conditions are hugely different. They also criticize the underlying assumptions of interprofessional collaboration that the patient is willing to take on the responsibilities that comes with being 'the centre of the team' and taking part in shared decision-making. According to Fox and Reeves (2015), shared decision-making is seen as a divestment of physician power and authority, both by the patients themselves and by other professions. We suggest that a competency domain of pedagogy and learning may be the possible missing link needed to articulate how interprofessional education to enhance learner outcomes is interdependent with collaborative practice to enhance patient outcomes.

One of the crucial points for the success of interprofessional education is the awareness of learners and teachers that interprofessional competence is not a separate capability. On the contrary, professional and interprofessional competences are inextricably intertwined. A crucial challenge is also to develop pedagogically engaged teachers. We believe that enhancing this awareness is necessary in order to maintain and improve the quality of the programmes and their delivery.

## Literature

Areskog N-H (2009). Undergraduate interprofessional education at the Linköping Faculty of Health Sciences - How it all started. *Journal of Interprofessional Care, 23*, 442-447.

Barr H, Koppel I, Reeves S, Hammick M, Freeth D (2005). *Effective interprofessional education: Argument, assumption and evidence.* Oxford: Blackwell.

Biggs JB & Tang CS (2011). *Teaching for quality learning at university: What the student does.* Maidenhead: Open University Press.

Boud D & Falchikov N (2006) Aligning assessment with long-term learning. *Assessment & Evaluation in Higher Education, 31*, 399–413.

Boud D, Thompson D & Lawson R (2013). Does student engagement in self-assessment calibrate their judgement over time? *Assessment and Evaluation In Higher Education, 38*, 941-956.

Buckley S, Coleman J, Davison I, Khan K, Zamora J, Malick S & ... Sayers J (2009). The educational effects of portfolios on undergraduate student learning: A Best Evidence Medical Education systematic review. *Medical Teacher, 31*, 340-355.

CAIPE (Centre for the Advancement of Interprofessional Education) (1997). *Interprofessional education – A definition.* CAIPE Bulletin 13, 19.

Dahlgren LO (2009). Interprofessional learning and problem-based learning – a marriage made in heaven? *Journal of Interprofessional Care, 23,* 448-54.

Ekeli B-V (2013). *Tvetydighet. En studie av samarbeid i helsetjenester og samarbeidslaering i helsepersonellutdanning.* Thesis. Norges Arktiske Universitet.

Faresjö T, Wilhelmsson M, Pelling S, Dahlgren L & Hammar M (2007). Does interprofessional education jeopardize medical skills? *Journal of Interprofessional Care, 21,* 573-576.

Fenwick T (2010). Rethinking the thing: Sociomaterial approaches to understanding and researching learning in work. *Journal of Workplace Learning 22,* 104-16.

Fox A & Reeves S (2015). Interprofessional collaborative patient-centred care: A critical exploration of two related discourses. *Journal of Interprofessional Care, 29,* 113-118.

Frenk, J, Chen L, Bhutta, Z, Cohen, J, Crisp N, Evans T, Fineberg H, Garcia P, Ke Y, Kelley P, Kistnasamy B, Meleis A, Naylor D, Pablos-Mendez A, Reddy S, Scrimshaw S, Sepulveda J, Serwadda D & Zurayk H (2010). Health professionals for a new century: Transforming education to strengthen health systems in an interdependent world. *Lancet, 376*, 1923-1958.

Hammar M, Bergdahl B & Öhman L (2006). *Celebrating the past by expanding the future: The Faculty of Health Sciences, Linköping University 1986–2006*. Linköping: Linköping University Electronic Press.

Interprofessional Education Collaborative Expert Panel (IPEC) (2011*). Core competencies for interprofessional collaborative practice: Report of an expert panel*. Washington, DC: Inter-professional Education Collaborative. Downloaded from https://www.aamc.org/download/ 186750/data/core_competencies.pdf

Lave J & Wenger E (1991). *Situated Learning. Legitimate peripheral participation.* Cambridge: University of Cambridge Press.

Lawlis TR, Anson J & Greenfield D (2014). Barriers and enablers that influence sustainable interprofessional education: A literature review. *Journal of Interprofessional Care, 28*, 305-310.

Lee A, Steketee C, Rogers G & Moran M (2013). Towards a theoretical framework for curriculum development in health professional education. *Focus On Health Professional Education, 14*, 70.

Lindh Falk A, Hult H, Hammar M, Hopwood N & Abrandt Dahlgren M (2013). One site fits all? A student ward as a learning practice for interprofessional development. *Journal of Interprofessional Care, 27*, 476-481.

Marton F, Hounsell D & Entwistle NJ (1998). *The experience of learning*. Edinburgh: Scottish Academic Press.

Norman GR & Schmidt HG (1992). The psychological bases of problem based learning: A review of the evidence. *Academic Medicine, 67*, 557-565.

Östergren J, Kaviani C, Thorvaldsen T, Krook-Brandt M & Dahlgren L-O (2009). Variation of internship test results depends on the seat of learning and age. Analysis of tests 1995-2008. *Läkartidningen, 106* (38), 2354-2356.

O'Sullivan A, Harris P, Hughes C, Jones P, Scicluna H, Howe A & ... Leinster S (2012). Does a summative portfolio foster the development of capabilities such as reflective practice and understanding ethics? An evaluation from two medical schools. *Medical Teacher, 34*, e21-e28.

Persson A, Fyrenius A, Bergdahl B (2010). Perspectives on using multimedia scenarios in a PBL medical curriculum. *Medical Teacher, 32*, 766-772.

Reeves S, Tassone M, Parker K, Wagner SJ & Simmons B (2012). Interprofessional education: An overview of key developments in the past three decades. *Work, 41*, 233-245.

Savery JR & Duffy TM (1995). Problem based learning: An instructional model and its constructivist framework. *Educational Technology, 35*, 31-7.

Schraw G (1998). Promoting general metacognitive awareness. *Instructional Science, 26*, 113-25.

Schön D (1987). *Educating the reflective practitioner*. San Francisco, CA: Jossey-Bass.

Säljö R (2000). *Lärande i praktiken. Ett sociokulturellt perspektiv.* Stockholm: Prisma.

Thistletwaite J (2012). Interprofessional education: A review of context, learning and the research agenda. *Medical Education, 46*, 58–70.

Wilhelmsson M (2011). *Developing interprofessional competence: Theoretical and empirical contributions.* (Doctoral dissertation). Linköping: Linköping University Electronic Press.

World Health Organisation (2010). *Framework for action on interprofessional education & collaborative practice.* Geneva: WHO Press.

For information on interprofessional practice and education in Europe, visit the website of the European Interprofessional Practice and Education Network (EIPEN):

www.eipen.eu

# Interprofessional education in health and social care: Changing students' opinions

Majda Pahor, Teja Škodič Zakšek, Renata Vettorazzi, Nevenka Ferfila and Matic Kavčič

## The cultural context of interprofessional collaboration in Slovenian health care

In the last two decades, Slovenia has experienced many political and social transformations which have had impact on the health care system, but it is difficult to say whether these have brought about more collaborative relationships. Some studies (Klemenc & Pahor 2001, Skela-Savič 2006) found that hierarchical relationships between different health professionals as well as between health professionals and users still persist. Another indicator of the cultural background that may inhibit collaboration is the level of social capital, measured as the level of generalized trust. In Slovenia, social capital is low compared to other European countries, and collaboration and integration inadequate at all levels of the social system (Delhey & Newton 2003, Iglič 2004). Slovenia belongs in the cultural and political space of predominantly Catholic Central Europe. According to Inglehart (1997), Catholic countries have lower levels of trust because of the hierarchical social structure, shaped by the Church. In these countries, religiosity is connected with value orientations characterised by obedience and subservience (Inglehart 1997).

In Slovenia, there has been little research into the relational aspects of health care, and specifically into interprofessional collaboration. There is lack of evidence but there are diverse anecdotal interpretations of the characteristics of collaboration, varying from critical examples of subordination and even abuse to idealized descriptions. So far only the relationships between nurses and doctors have been systematically studied. A multi method study, including surveys, interviews and observational studies was conducted between 2005 and 2009. The study started with a survey of a national sample of nurses and doctors, complemented with interviews with study participants, followed by a survey of nursing and medical students, observational case study research in clinical practice and ethnography with participant observation (Kvas e.a. 2006, Pahor 2008).

Findings showed that the participants hold different profession-related attitudes towards collaboration, and, as indicated in the observational studies, there were even more differences in experiencing collaboration in practice. Doctors mainly saw collaboration with nurses as unproblematic, while nurses expressed more critical views. Such differences are not a good starting point for developing successful team work and collaboration. On the other hand, there were significant similarities between the two professions indicating a common culture of readiness to work together, a high appreciation of the other profession, and a knowledge about the roles of both professions. Expressing disagreement in work situations was a problem for all the included professions.

The research showed a less than satisfactory situation in relation to collaboration, and the next step of the project group of clinicians and academics was to introduce developments to bring about at least more collaborative attitudes in future health care in Slovenia. The change that the educators can introduce, is a new way of preparing future health professionals for their work, by developing relevant courses and offering students interprofessional learning opportunities.

## The development of interprofessional education in Slovenia

So far, two interprofessional courses in health and social care have been developed and implemented in Slovenia. The first was an international, interprofessional and IT supported course in palliative care for Slovenian and Swedish students, called *Dying and mourning*, developed in collaboration between University of Ljubljana and University of Umea, Sweden. The collaboration included the two project leaders, students from six different health care disciplines in both countries and experts in the field. The idea for the project was to develop a student centred, IT-supported interdisciplinary and international course in palliative care, the working language being English. Students from both countries participated in the development of the course. Their own experiences of good and bad death were the starting point for planning the teaching session, and in the individual work phase students determined their own pace and time of study. Students entered discussions with each other and with course leaders at the time of their convenience. The course ran as an elective between 2001 and 2008 (Pahor & Rasmussen 2009).

On the basis of experiences from this international IPE course, and as a response to identified needs for IP education, an elective course at the Faculty of Health Studies at Ljubljana University was developed called *Interprofessional collaboration in health care teams*. The course is offered to the students of most of its departments (nursing, midwifery, physiotherapy, occupational therapy, sanitary engineering, radiography) and to students from three other faculties: medicine, social work and psychology. The course is run by an interprofessional teaching team of 10 teachers with varied professional background: nursing, occupational therapy, physical therapy, radiography, sanitary engineering, midwifery, sociology, psychology, social work and medicine.

The course has been organised as a 6 credits, lasting for four months with a combination of lectures, seminars and small group work both in classroom and in virtual space. It is structured in two parts, called respectively "Gaining strengths" and "Facing the problem". The whole teaching and learning process is supported by virtual class-room on the platform Moodle where all the information about the course and about the participants are accessible together with learning materials, guidelines and instructions for their assignments. It includes the course syllabus as accredited at the University of Ljubljana, the course information package for students, the outline and description of the lectures, guidelines for students' mid-course paper, and guidelines for the seminar work, for the teamwork on the patient's problems as well as for the final rapport. Students' work assessment criteria are included. There are also information on forms and procedures of course evaluation. A teachers' manual, prepared by the course leader and discussed and improved during each teachers' team meeting with the exact plan to carry out the course helps the teaching team to hold together. It contains also the guidelines for the teachers in relation to the aims of the course. Keeping the red line of the course is a demanding task for all the teachers and for the course leader, as the participating teachers have many other obligations which interfere with involvement in this course. However, the teachers try to set an example of good team work to the students by their own engagement and efficient collaboration.

Aims of the course are that the students gain knowledge about the roles and scope of practice of different professions, about complementarity of their competencies and become able to plan and carry out team work in relation to patients' problems.

In the first part of the course, "Gaining strengths", the main aims are to enable the students to learn about the competences and scope of practice of all the professions involved, and about the advantages and risks of the teamwork. The teaching methods here include lectures, seminar group work and home work individual assignments. Lectures are given by the members of the teaching team and some invited speakers, for example representatives of patients associations.

The connection between the lectures for the whole class and seminar work in smaller groups is a paper that students prepare on the basis of the lectures and the literature study. By answering guiding questions, they demonstrate their knowledge of teamwork as well as the roles of different professions and health care users.

Seminar work is organised in three parts:

A. Knowledge about the professions, the users and teamwork (recognizing elements of team work, problems with team functioning and team development strategies)
B. Advantages and risks of working with differences: professions related stereotypes and prejudices, stereotypes about patients, media images of health professions, users and their relations
C. Teamwork exercises: of self-presentation, of trust, of collaboration, and task-related

Post-exercise reflection is crucial to success – sharing experiences, doubts, comments is a part of the team formation, and an opportunity to knowing personal sides of team members. One important exercise is role-swapping – students play the role of another profession and are assessed by the respective profession.

In the second part, "Facing the problem", students work in teams with a health care user. This part takes 2-3 weeks and enables students to bring together all the knowledge from earlier parts of the course to apply to problems – both concerning functioning as a team and solving patients' problems. During this period teachers as well as practitioners provide help if needed. In their final report, the students present not only the patients' problems and the team suggestions for the patients, but also the team development process, any problems they have faced and how they have dealt with them. A reflection on the whole interprofessional experience concludes the paper. The papers are published on the course IT platform, read and commented on by other students and teachers, and presented in seminar groups. After the comments are received, students rework their final reports and hand them in for the summative assessment, based on content-related and formal criteria, published on the course website.

To support students' learning, the teaching team wrote a course text book, *Partners for health: Interprofessional collaboration* (Pahor 2014). This is organised in three sections. The first introduces interprofessional collaboration in health care, its background, reasons for and barriers against, as well as different types of teams and their functioning. The second part presents the partners for health: health care users and different professionals. The first chapter is a sociological view of the role and position of health care users, including a literature review and some excerpts from actual research on users' voice in Slovenia. The following chapters concern the competences and roles of 9 professions: nursing, physiotherapy, occupational therapy, radiography, sanitary engineering, midwifery, medicine, psychology and social work. The third section is focused on developing team work skills and is more practically oriented, and intended to be used in class or during lifelong education, and includes patients' cases. The book was written to help the actual and future health professionals in Slovenia to develop respectful and efficient collaboration, both with other professionals and with the users. It gives information about the diversity of competences in health care and their possible synergetic effects through collaborative team work.

## Experiences and dilemmas of first implementations

In the process of the course development we have prepared several monitoring instruments to gather information about the needs for such a course, as well as to establish ways of evaluating our work and the outcome. Our main aim was to evaluate the short-term influence of the IP course on student opinion and knowledge about different aspects of interprofessional education and practice. However our ambition is to develop a panel study that will provide deeper under-standing of the long-lasting effects of IP education. We present here some preliminary results of the gathered data.

We have used various methods to generate a source of qualitative and quantitative data. The need for the course among students was tested by a pre-course anonymous open-ended questionnaire testing initial knowledge about participating professions (carried out in 2011-2012, N=73). Student opinions on various aspects of IPE were gathered with the adapted Bristol questionnaire (Pollard e.a. 2004; Peterle 2006). Student opinions were measured by 9 items (on a four-point scale) immediately before the beginning of the course and immediately after the end of the course. In the first two years PAPI (pen-and-paper interviewing) questionnaires were administered among the participating students, later an online survey was designed with the same survey questions. However the survey was expanded in 2014-2015 by another set of questions in order to enable future investigations. The response rate was relatively high (78% out of 239 students, 79% for the pre-test and 77% for the post-test) and the analysed samples were as follows: in 2011/12, pre-test N=64, post-test N=73, in 2012/13, pre-test N=50, post-test N=53, in 2013/14 pre-test N=34, post-test N=25, in 2014/2015 pre-test N=40, post-test N=32. Independent sample T-test was used to compare means between student opinions. Due to imperfect coding of the PAPI questionnaires in the first two years we could not match pre-test and post-test answers of the respondents. Thus the analysis presented here could only be calculated at the aggregate level. Further limitations apply since although there was approximately half a year between the measurements they are not independent. In the future repeated measures ANOVA will be performed. Qualitative thematic analysis of open-ended questionnaire was used to investigate initial understanding of other professions and to analyse an open-ended survey question: How would you define the term "health care team"? The answers were coded in Atlas.ti.

## Initial understanding of other professions

In order to gain insight into students' initial knowledge about other professions we have asked them to describe midwifery, occupational therapy, physiotherapy, radiologic technology, sanitary engineering, nursing and health psychology. This was our simple needs assessment tool which would guide the content of the first part of the course (*gaining strengths*). We have come across some disappointing results, especially considering that all the participating students were in their final year and will soon start their professional career. The knowledge about other professions was poor. Students' answers frequently contained wrong descriptions and were often on the level of stereotypes. They used lay terminology and focused their descriptions around the working tasks instead of professions. Stereotypical understanding of midwifery, nursing and physiotherapy was the most prominent, as these two illustrative examples demonstrate:

> Midwifery: *"Vocation, of mostly women, who care for the newborns and help during the delivery."*

> Physiotherapy: *"This is an area that deals with massage and tries to eliminate pain in muscles and skeleton with massage."*

On the other hand we have evidence of the poorest knowledge of occupational therapy, sanitary engineering, radiologic technology and health psychology.

> Radiologic technology: *"Deals with apparatus in operating rooms, identifies signs, reads functions from the apparatus by the patient's bed."*

> Occupational therapy: *"An occupational therapist deals with illness and injuries sustained at the workplace. He tries to remove or lessen injuries to the acceptable level." "Healing, rehabilitation with handcrafts."*

Whereas the lack of knowledge about health psychology was expected (since the programme is running in another faculty), findings on other professions were unexpected. However there were also some examples of good knowledge such as:

> Nursing: *"Profession that deals with the care of the patient on all 14 basic life activities. Takes care of promotion, support and health recovery."*

These results demonstrated a lack of understanding of roles of different professions, thus revealing a gap and deficiency of respective study programs and a need for such a course. Finally the course provided and tested different forms of knowledge (in the form of homework assignments and final report) about other professions. Up till now all the students who attended the full course successfully completed it.

## IP course impact on student opinions

A range of statements on various aspects of IPE were included in the survey to test students' initial opinions and possibly a change in their opinions that could be ascribed to the experience of the IP course. The answers were given on a four-point scale from 1 (strongly agree) to 4 (strongly disagree). The results are shown in tables below. Based on these results it can be speculated that the students who enlisted in this elective course were already inclined to IPE and opened to teamwork as the averages (between agree and strongly agree) of pre-test measurement on statements expressing positive opinion on IPE imply. On a 4-point scale however there was little room for improvement. Nonetheless, on average the impact of the course on all statements seem to have caused even more positive IPE opinions and some of the changes were statistically significant.

On the basis of these results it seems that the impact of our course did leave some positive effects on the opinions of the students towards IPE and IP collaboration. However the changes were small and only some were statistically significant. With the help of several evaluation tools the team of teachers tried to evolve and improve the course during the years. There were some changes such as introduction of 'alive patients' instead of paper cases in 2013/14, inclusion of medical students in 2014/15, and modification of teamwork exercises which might have affected the results. However this would need to be studied in more detail in future. Nevertheless it seems the improvement is visible especially between the first year which was understandably full of teething problems and the second year. In the end we have to again emphasise that this is an elective course thus we can speculate the impact would have been greater for those students with less positive initial opinions towards IPE and less opened to IP collaboration and teamwork, who might profit more.

At the end of the survey an open-ended question measured students' understanding of the "health care team" before and after the course. Again we discovered there was already good initial understanding of the concept. The majority of answers used the following terms to describe the health care team: group (of) various experts (who) collaborate (with) a common goal for the benefit of the patient. After the IP course the students gave more elaborate answers. They have mentioned more often a holistic approach, common goals, shared decision-making, equal role of the team members, mutual understanding and respect. The descriptions included the organisation and coordination through mutual adjustment, the benefits of complementing each other, and the importance to expand and share the knowledge for better results. Importantly elements of user (and family) involvement (such as active, patient-centred approach, patient's needs, patient's problems, patient as a team member) were mentioned more often.

Table 6: Student opinions on various aspects of IPE before and after the IP course.

| Year / N | Measurement | Mean | SD | t | p |
|---|---|---|---|---|---|
| *My skills in communicating with patients would be improved through this learning.* | | | | | |
| 2011- / 63 | Before | 2,06 | 0,592 | 0,462 | 0,645 |
| 2012 / 73 | After | 2,01 | 0,656 | | |
| 2012- / 50 | Before | 2,14 | 0,639 | 2,444 | 0,016 |
| 2013 / 53 | After | 1,85 | 0,568 | | |
| 2013- / 34 | Before | 2,26 | 0,666 | 1,536 | 0,130 |
| 2014 / 25 | After | 2,00 | ,645 | | |
| 2014- / 40 | Before | 2,40 | 1,033 | 1,62 | 0,110 |
| 2015 / 32 | After | 2,03 | 0,861 | | |
| *This learning is likely to facilitate professional relations.* | | | | | |
| 2011- / 63 | Before | 1,84 | 0,574 | 2,68 | 0,008 |
| 2012 / 73 | After | 1,59 | 0,523 | | |
| 2012- / 50 | Before | 1,80 | 0,571 | 3,075 | 0,003 |
| 2013 / 53 | After | 1,45 | 0,574 | | |
| 2013- / 34 | Before | 1,74 | 0,618 | 0,480 | 0,633 |
| 2014 / 25 | After | 1,64 | 0,907 | | |
| 2014- / 40 | Before | 1,73 | 0,599 | 1,69 | 0,095 |
| 2015 / 32 | After | 1,50 | 0,508 | | |
| *This learning would likely improve my teamwork skills.* | | | | | |
| 2011- / 64 | Before | 1,80 | 0,568 | 1,94 | 0,054 |
| 2012 / 73 | After | 1,62 | 0,517 | | |
| 2012- / 50 | Before | 1,84 | 0,650 | 3,132 | 0,002 |
| 2013 / 53 | After | 1,47 | 0,541 | | |
| 2013- / 34 | Before | 1,91 | 0,621 | 1,108 | 0,274 |
| 2014 / 25 | After | 1,68 | 0,900 | | |
| 2014- / 40 | Before | 1,73 | 0,599 | 1,13 | 0,263 |
| 2015 / 32 | After | 1,56 | 0,619 | | |
| *This learning is likely to help to overcome stereotypes about different professions.* | | | | | |
| 2011- / 64 | Before | 1,78 | 0,678 | 1,97 | 0,050 |
| 2012 / 73 | After | 1,56 | 0,623 | | |
| 2012- / 50 | Before | 1,90 | 0,614 | 3,593 | 0,001 |
| 2013 / 53 | After | 1,49 | 0,541 | | |
| 2013- / 33 | Before | 1,73 | 0,674 | 1,090 | 0,280 |
| 2014 / 25 | After | 1,52 | 0,770 | | |
| 2014- / 40 | Before | 1,65 | 0,580 | 0,40 | 0,692 |
| 2015 / 32 | After | 1,59 | 0,615 | | |

Scale: 1 – strongly agree, 2 – agree, 3 – disagree, 4 – strongly disagree

Based on these preliminary findings we are confident that we have filled the gap in knowledge about other professions and changed some views and opinions on IPE. We have also tackled some stereotypes about teamwork of health care workers. However, greater and deeper understanding of IPE and IP collaboration is needed. Future research will show whether or not the results suggested here are only short-term or whether the IPE has enduring and lasting effects. Therefore our challenge for the future is to conduct a panel or cohort study and evolve the course further according to its results possibly also in the clinical settings.

## Conclusions: which way forward?

The process of development and accreditation of this inter-faculty course at Ljubljana University unravelled some contextual barriers. Ljubljana University is a very loosely connected association of 25 faculties and three art academies with great autonomy and differences in educational philosophy and practice. Also, the idea of inter-faculty elective courses has not settled down completely and encounters huge problems of embedding such courses in different professions' curricula. Challenges for the future are to introduce team work learning in the clinical settings and to bring students into real life of existing teams in health care. Another aspect which needs careful consideration is the cultural setting of the Slovenian health care. Its values, beliefs, and norms influence health professionals' performance and behaviour.

The students and teachers involved in the teaching and learning process need a reflection of their own positions and roles to respond to their curiosity, initiative, and readiness to change and develop. The active involvement of patients as collaborators and teachers to students also demand additional engagement. In times of cuttings in the public sector, faculties are understaffed, and existing teachers' workloads don't encourage developing innovative teaching and learning approaches.

## Literature

Delhey J & Newton K (2003). Who trusts? The origins of social trust in seven societies. *European Societies, 5, 93-138.*

Iglič H (2004). Dejavniki nizke stopnje zaupanja v Sloveniji/Determinants of the low level of trust in Slovenia. *Družboslovne razprave, 20, 149-175.*

Inglehardt R (1997). *Modernization and postmodernization: Cultural, economic and political change in 43 societies.* Princeton, New Jersey: Princeton University Press.

Klemenc D & Pahor M (Eds.) (2001). *Medicinske sestre v Sloveniji: zbornik člankov s Strokovnega srečanja z mednarodno udeležbo.* Ljubljana: Društvo medicinskih sester in zdravstvenih tehnikov/*Nurses in Slovenia: papers from international conference.* Ljubljana: Nursing and Nursing Assistants Association.

Kvas A, Pahor M, Klemenc D, Šmitek J (Eds.) (2006). *Sodelovanje med medicinskimi sestrami in zdravniki v zdravstvenem timu: priložnost za izboljšanje kakovosti*

*[Collaboration between nurses and doctors in health care teams: An opportunity to improve quality]*. Ljubljana: Nursing and Nursing Assistants Association.

Pahor M (2008). Interprofessional relationships: Doctors and nurses in Slovenia. In E Kuhlmann & M Saks (Eds.). *Rethinking professional governance: International directions in health care*. Bristol: Policy.

Pahor M & Rasmussen B (2009). How does culture show? A case study of an international and interprofessional course in palliative care. *Journal of Interprofessional Care, 23*, 474-485.

Pahor M (Ed.) (2014). *Zavezniki za zdravje: medpoklicno sodelovanje v zdravstvenih timih*. Zdravstvena fakulteta *[Partners for health: Interprofessional collaboration in health care teams]*. Ljubljana: Faculty of Health Sciences.

Peterle H (2006). Stališča študentov medicine in zdravstvene nege Univerze v Ljubljani do medpoklicnega sodelovanja [Attitudes of nursing and medical students of Ljubljana University about interprofessional collaboration]. *Obzornik zdravstvene nege, 40*, 129-136.

Pollard KC, Miers ME & Gilchrist M (2004). Collaborative learning for collaborative working? Initial findings from a longitudinal study of health and social care students. *Health and Social Care in the Community, 12*, 346–358.

Skela-Savič B (2006) Organisational culture in Slovene hospitals. In *Advancing business and management in knowledge-based society - Proceedings of the 7th International Conference of the Faculty of Management, University of Primorska, 23-25 November 2006, Portorož, Slovenia*. Koper: Faculty of Management.

# The development and implementation of an interprofessional study programme: A multifaceted approach

Anita Stevens, Albine Moser and Sandra Beurskens

## The setting in the Netherlands

The number of elderly people and people with multiple chronic diseases increases worldwide. In the Netherlands it is estimated that in 2025 about 25% of the people will be aged 65 and older (Garssen 2011). In order to deal with the complex healthcare demands of these people, professionals from the different disciplines have to collaborate. The World Health Organisation (WHO 2010) and Freek and colleagues (2010) advocate interprofessional education (IPE) to prepare the future health professionals to learn how to work together in order to tackle those health care challenges.

For this reason IPE has become a policy spearhead of the Faculty of Health at Zuyd University of applied sciences. The Faculty has the ambition of educating students to become critical and innovative health care professionals. To prepare future professionals, students must have the competences needed to work together with other professions.

Zuyd University of Applied Science (Zuyd) is located in three different cities of the southern province of the Netherlands: Heerlen, Maastricht and Sittard. The Faculty of Healthcare is located in the city of Heerlen and Maastricht and hosts educational programmes and research centres. The study programmes are: occupational therapy, speech and language therapy, physiotherapy, nursing, arts therapy, biomedical technologies, and midwifery. There are approximately 1500 students and 260 educators.

The aim of this chapter is to provide insights into the development and the implementation of IPE over a four-year period from the beginning in 2011. While walking along it we were also creating the road of IPE. In this sense, we describe the IPE working group, the systematic approach and the developed implementation strategies. We also highlight our reflections on the most significant experiences and challenges.

## The IP working group: A systematic approach

In order to develop interprofessional education (IPE), an interprofessional working group, called 'IPOS' (in Dutch: Inter-Professioneel Opleiden en Samenwerken [Interprofessional Education and Collaboration]) was initiated in November 2011. The task of the group was to develop a shared framework for interprofessional collaboration and to model and structure IPE in the curricula of seven health programmes and social work. Eight professionals with different background in one IP working group was the beginning of challenging and intensive collaboration in an interprofesional team. An advantage was that the education system of all the participating education programmes is based on the Problem Based Learning system (Neville 2009), a student-based pedagogy where students work together in mono-disciplinary tutorial groups. We thought this shared concept would facilitate the design and implementation of an IPE programme and interprofessional collaboration among educators. When we started our assumption was that we 'only' had to cross the interprofessional boundaries of the educators.

We chose to work systematically and stepwise as in an implementation process. We chose the model of Grol and colleagues (2005, 2013) to guide our implementation. In this five-step model changes in healthcare are implemented in an efficient way (see Figure 10). We considered that changing an educational system at faculty level needs behaviour change of all educators, and that working together in the IP working group to design and implement IPE is similar to working together in a healthcare team. Implementation is an ongoing cyclical process and is not a chronological process where the different steps as the description implies follow each other in a logical order. Rather, we used it as a guiding model.

First we developed and defined the IPE programme as a proposal for change. Next we analysed the setting (in our case seven educational programmes at the faculty of Healthcare and Social work) in which the IPE had to be implemented. We also studied enablers and barriers. Then we developed multifaceted implementation strategies that would be piloted and evaluated and subsequently readjusted. During the implementation process we considered the phases in a process of change (Grol & Wensing 2004). In this chapter we describe the first three steps of the implementation model.

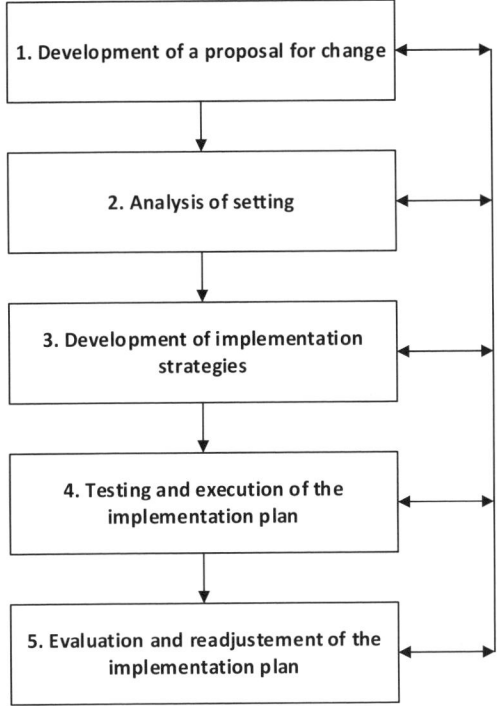

Figure 10: Implementation model of Grol e.a. (2005, 2013).

## Step 1: The development of a proposal for change

The proposal for change was the IPE programme. The development of this IPE programme was based on several basic principles. These were: a shared vision, a common language, and a shared framework of interprofessional competences. These principles described below were conceived by the IP working group as a prerequisite to work together as a team and to implement the IPE programme.

### A shared vision

Because we had previous experiences with a three- month multidisciplinary module ten years before, we used our knowledge from this experience and formulated a shared vision for the new IPE programme. The shared vision started with the following agreed starting points, IPE has to: 1) be well integrated in the existing curricula, 2) be well balanced in relation to the specific professional competencies, 3) start in year one of every educational programme, and 4) involve the curriculum committee of every educational programme to support the development and implementation of the IPE programme.

The IP working group chose shared definitions of central concepts. For IPE we used the WHO definition of IPE: "Interprofessional Education occurs when two or more professionals learn about, from and with each other to come to enable collaboration and improve health outcomes" (WHO 2010). We also agreed on a shared vision of client-centred care since this was considered as the key purpose of IPE and we adapted the five conceptual dimensions as described by Mead and Bower (2000): biopsychosocial perspective, `patient-as-person', sharing power and responsibility, therapeutic alliance, and `doctor-as-person'.

## A common language

We experienced a lot of misunderstandings in our IP working group meetings due to language problems. As different educators with different professional backgrounds and working methods, we were often talking in different professional languages about the same issues or terms. For example, depending on the profession, the terms care plan, treatment plan, intervention plan or activity plan were used. We experienced that we were talking on different levels and sometimes really could not understand each other. In this phase, a lot of discussions took place and we did not make much progress. We had to learn to listen to each other, to accept the differences and to trust each other. We therefore decided to use a shared terminology. The International Classification of Functioning (ICF) (WHO 2001) was chosen because it was known by most educators and integrated in several educational programmes. The ICF is a classification system to describe all relevant aspects of human functioning in different domains (see Figure 11).

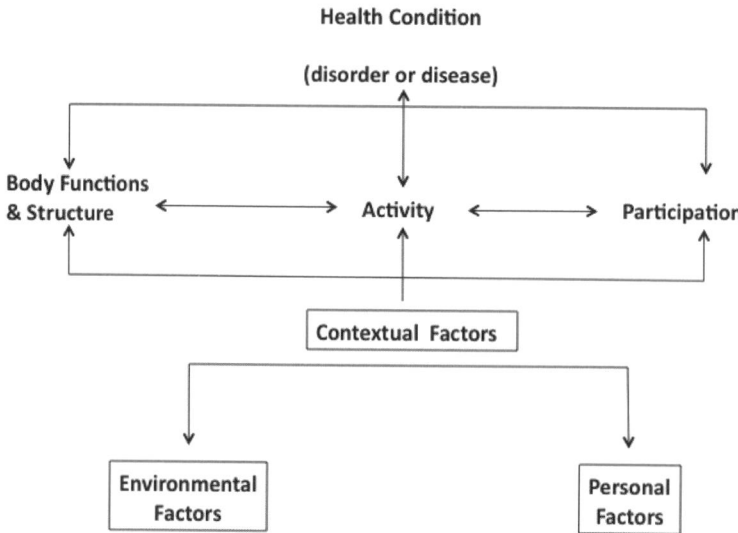

Figure 11: The ICF model.

## A shared framework of interprofessional competences

For the development of a shared framework of interprofessional competences we undertook a literature study. The framework was built upon several existing models and competences, in which the competence model of Hugh Barr (1998) was used as a starting point (Figure 12). This model describes the competences every healthcare professional should have acquired: common, complementary and collaborative competences. Common means competences held in common between all professions. Complementary means competences, which distinguish one profession and complement those that distinguish other professions.

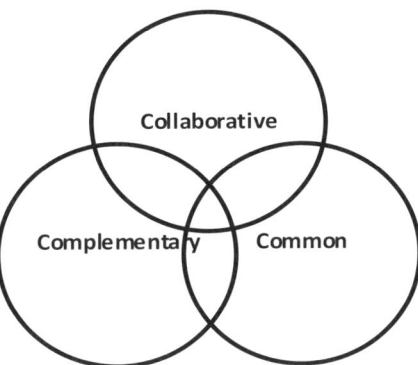

Figure 12: Competence model by Barr (1998).

Collaborative means dimensions of competence which every profession needs to collaborate within its own ranks, with other professions, with non-professionals, within organisations, between organisations, with patients and their caregivers, with volunteers and with community groups.

To define the collaborative competences in more detail we used the five interprofessional key competences identified by Vyt (2009, see Figure 13):

- Consult and collaborate effectively in IP teams, on the basis of knowledge of competences of healthcare workers;
- Work out patient-centred shared care plans on the basis of information and interaction with other healthcare workers;
- Anticipate, identify and remediate problems in IP teamwork and shared care planning;
- Make appropriate referrals to other healthcare workers based on the knowledge of competences of healthcare workers;
- Evaluate IP communication, decision making and care planning in terms of efficiency.

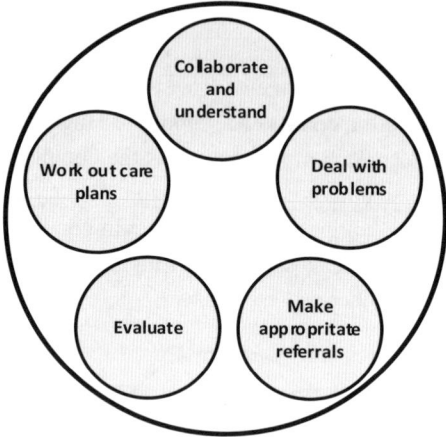

Figure 13: Interprofessional key competences (Vyt, 2009).

Additionally, the CanMed roles (Frank 2005) of professional, scholar, manager, expert, health advocate, communicator and team player were integrated because most healthcare professions in the Netherlands adapted these roles in their (revised) professional competence framework and also guided the educational programme. We placed the role of collaborator (Barr 1998) and the five key IP competences (Vyt 2009) at the centre of the CanMed roles. The integration of these three models formed the 'Zuyd IPE competence model' (see Figure 14).

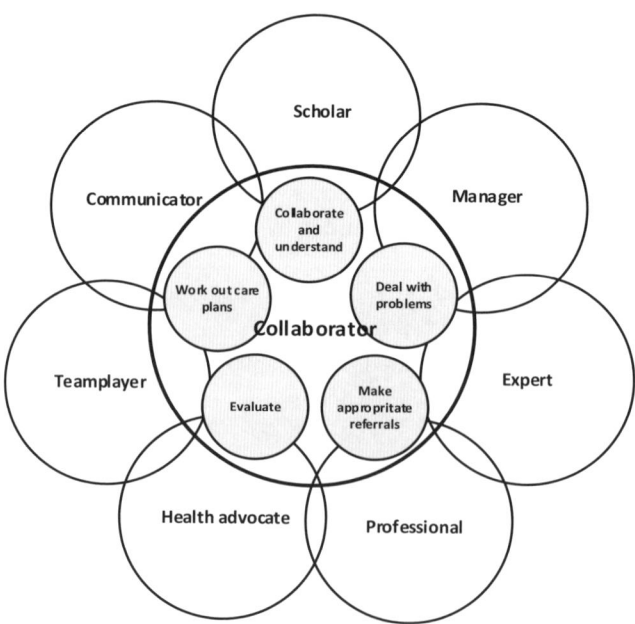

Figure 14: Integration of models into the 'Zuyd IPE competence model'.

In the next step we started to develop descriptors for all of the five key competencies which resulted in 39 separate descriptors. This process was carried out by three members of the working group and subsequently discussed in working sessions with all members of the working group, until consensus was reached. We also checked if these descriptors fitted to the content of all educational programmes.

To implement the interprofessional competences in the different curriculum designs, we organised two interactive working sessions within our IP working group. In these sessions we discussed, refined and finally agreed to order the descriptors of the IP competences in different levels. In this way we were able to serve all the study programmes. The 39 descriptors were ranged in terms of complexity, transferability and responsibility according to the Dublin descriptors (Joint Quality Initiative Informal Group 2004) and the Dutch version of the European Qualification Framework (Adviescommissie NLQF–EQ 2011). According to the Dublin descriptors we arranged the levels as 1a and 1b as beginner, level 2 as medium and level 3a and 3b as the exit level. The exit level is equivalent to level 6 of the European Qualification Framework. Our final product was a shared framework of IP competences and descriptors in different levels to cover the whole bachelor programme: the Zuyd IPE building blocks. In this process of developing a shared framework of interprofessional competencies, the curriculum committees of all education programmes were involved and regularly informed about the progress that was made.

## Step 2: Analysis of the Zuyd University setting

Important steps for implementation are to get to know the setting in which the proposal for change, in our case the new IPE programme, has to be implemented as well as analyses of facilitators and barriers.

### The setting
To get to know the setting we analysed the existing IPE activities in the curricula of the eight educational programmes. We explored which IPE elements already were present and which could be further developed. We drew up an inventory for all of the curricula. Examples of existing IPE activities were: teachers from one educational programme giving lectures, workshops or demonstrations in other programmes. More specifically: a nurse gave a lecture about diabetes care or an occupational therapist demonstrated wheelchairs in physiotherapy. Also students were involved in IPE, for example speech therapy students played simulation patient with aphasia in the training of communication skills in physiotherapy. Students from different studies also worked together in different tutorial groups in the multi professional minor programmes, programmes that are offered in the optional study hours. In addition, a one-time educational event for all students in the faculty of Healthcare was the annual Patient Contact Day. Here students were assigned to

interprofessional groups and met patients to discuss their needs and problems in living with a chronic illness. In some study tasks and learning goals, interprofessional elements were integrated and the multi professional contribution to specific cases discussed and explored.

This inventory of the setting revealed the following points. A lot of IPE elements were already integrated into the curricula, which is positive. On the other hand, these IPE elements were very fragmented, more by-accident than in an organised way and they were often related to informal contact between educators . These IPE activities were also limited to knowledge transfer: it was more learning about each other and less from or with each other. In this way students learned little collaborative competencies. Furthermore, these IPE activities were not explicitly mentioned or identified in the curricula. It was a hidden element and the focus on the importance of IPE was lacking.

## Analysis of facilitators and barriers

The analysis of facilitators and barriers was done on different levels. The facilitators at the level of *individual educators* were: the urge to develop and implement IPE, personal motivation and a lot of enthusiasm. At *group level* (IP working group and curriculum committee) facilitators were: willingness to innovate, open and honest interaction, and readiness to collaborate. At *organisational level* facilitators were that the director supported the IP project group by assigning extra working hours to it, the vice-director advocated and supported IPE in the management team, and all but one educational programme were about to start re-designing their curricula.

Barriers at the *individual level* were: using different profession-specific languages, little interest in faculty development activities and defending professional boundaries. The most perceived barrier were time constraints experienced by each individual educator, due to several claims on them: regular teaching activities versus IPE activities. At the *group level* barriers were: little knowledge of each other's educational programmes, working in knowledge 'silo's', much turnover of members of the IP working group with the consequence that discussions started all over repeatedly, and different curriculum designs. At *organisational level* the main barrier centred on logistics and differing student schedules. In general, the attitude of most educators at the beginning was: 'you can never organise IPE across educational programmes'.

# Step 3: Development of implementation strategies

Parallel to the analysis of the Zuyd setting, we searched for best practice in IPE in the national and international literature and through contacting our (inter)national partner universities. These examples were used to develop the content of our IPE programme and adapted to the context of Zuyd. For example, we have good contacts with Robert Gordon University in Aberdeen, Scotland and Alesund University College in Norway. We consider them as our role models and contact them regularly. Based on the analysis of the setting and the facilitators and barriers as well as the information from the best practices, the following strategies for the implementation of the IPE programme were developed.

- Collaborative educational practice: As IPE is one of the spearheads of our faculty, interprofessional collaboration should also become a part of the teaching culture in the development and implementation of the IPE programme itself. Therefore, in all IPE teaching activities two or more educators from different educational programmes work together to develop, execute, evaluate and improve IPE activities.
- Start with 'low hanging fruit' and small opportunities: We encouraged our working group members to initiate and carry out small and easy-to-implement IPE activities. We agreed that every educational programme should work out a plan for at least one new small-scale IPE activity a year. For example, bio-medical technologies invited nursing students as simulation patients while performing ECGs. In order to learn from each other the nursing students also provided feedback to biomedical technology students on how patient-centred the communication with them was during the ECG exercise. In order to learn to know each other and to learn about each other's profession, we added a small exercise to the existing programme of the annual Patient Contact Day.
- Involving partners: IPE should involve all relevant stakeholders. We continuously involved educators from all educational programmes in our IP working group. In a later phase, a representative of the House of Care, a patient umbrella organisation, became involved as a permanent member. Also, students from all educational programmes and partners from health care institutions have been involved in yearly IPE think tanks. These think tanks provide valuable input to develop and implement IPE.
- Continuing exchange with the management team: The vice-director participated at all meetings with the curriculum committee. He was also involved in the team leaders meetings. He is the communication channel and linking-pin between policy, management, curriculum committee and IP working group. In this way fast communications, rapid responses and interactive feedback loops were possible.
- Faculty development for IPE: We started providing workshops for educators and at a later phase, we used informal learning as strategy, educators were teaching IPE in peer-pairs.
- Zuyd IPE building blocks: We asked the curriculum committees to approve these and commit to them. The Zuyd IPE building blocks were at the basis of our IPE activities and are referred to in unit books and teachers manuals.

- IPE pathway based on Zuyd IPE building blocks: The Zuyd IPE building blocks have been used to develop a four-year IPE pathway. Year 1 has been piloted and evaluated; year 2 is under development and will be implemented in the next academic year. Years 3 and 4 will be developed and implemented subsequently.
- Flexible logistics: We encouraged flexible teaching schedules across administrative boundaries and looked for logistical solutions such as IPE activities at the early evening (availability of sufficient teaching classes).
- Mixing and matching learning methods: IPE used a variety of learning and teaching methods: workshops, interactive demonstrations, lectures, skills trainings, learning tasks etc.
- Large-scale and sustainable implementation: We agreed on with the curriculum committees that IPE would be integrated in a coherent manner in all curricula during the curriculum re-design. This means: assigning credits (1 credit per academic year in all educational programmes), IPE obligatory for all students, integration in the regulatory bodies by the examination boards, and providing a 'special earmark' at the bachelor's diploma when students have earned all four credits for IPE.
- IP community of practices: We plan to expand our IP communities of practice further by involving Zuyd, patient organisations, students and health care institutions.

We used the phases in a process of change (Grol & Wensing 2004) to guide the development and implementation of IPE: orientation, insight, acceptance, change and preservation of change. A few examples of how we met the different levels are described in Table 7.

For example, in the first workshops for educators we especially addressed the behavioural aspects of orientation (promote awareness) and insight (create understanding). Also, we published short educational notes about IPE in our faculty newsletter and we gave short informative presentations to all educators in all programmes. To increase acceptance (develop a positive attitude) we worked with 'low hanging fruit' and small opportunities strategy especially to earn quick gains. We developed the Zuyd IPE building blocks and we involved relevant stakeholders in a dialogical manner. To initiate change (change practice) we looked for flexible and in particular, pragmatic logistical solutions and started to develop and implement the IPE pathway (IPE in year 1). To preserve change (integrate new practices into routine) we made agreements with the curriculum committees about large-scale implementation and sustainability (ECs), as well as developing the IP communities of practice. At the beginning we focused in the implementation of our strategies by involving students, educators and the curriculum committees. Team leaders, patients and health care institutions join at a later point of time.

Table 7: Model for the process of change (Grol & Wensing 2004) including the Zuyd implementation strategies.

| Stage of behaviour change | Implementation goals | Implementation strategies |
| --- | --- | --- |
| Orientation | Creating awareness, interest and involvement | Workshop with educators<br>Short educational notes in faculty newsletter<br>Informative presentations |
| Insight | Increasing knowledge and understanding | Workshop with educators<br>Short educational notes in faculty newsletter<br>Informative presentations |
| Acceptance | Positive attitude and motivation<br>Intention and decision to change | Involving partners<br>Low hanging fruits<br>Small opportunities<br>Zuyd IPE building blocks<br>Exchange with management team |
| Change | Implementation in daily practice | Logistical solutions<br>IPE pathway<br>Mixing and matching learning methods |
| Preservation of change | Integration in daily routines<br>Anchoring in the organisation | 4 credits obligatory in every educational programme<br>Integration in education- and examination regulatory body<br>'Special earmark' on diplomas<br>IP community of practice |

# Looking back and next steps forward: Lessons learned

We started in 2011 and in the past four years we learned a lot about, from and with each other in our IP working group. We developed as a team and started forming an IP community of practice. We now consider the Zuyd IPE competence model as our basic framework. The most important element in the implementation and development of IPE is at the outset to take time for the creation of a shared vision and starting points. The introduction of Barr's model (1998), with the common, collaborative and complementary competences took away much of the resistance of our colleagues. In the beginning they feared that there was not enough space for their own profession specific (complementary) competences in IPE.

An important lesson was that we had to pay attention to our own collaborative competences. We had to start with 'getting to know each other' on many occasions. We learned that this was absolutely necessary for creating a safe environment to enable crossing borders and finding common ground. The most striking experience in the first meetings with the curriculum committees was that they had to work through the same issues such as non-understanding and speaking other professional languages, as our IP working group did. We learned that this was an inevitable process that could not be skipped or accelerated. This process reflects the first stages of behaviour change: awareness and insight. Being occupied with our assignment, sometimes we were two steps ahead of the educators and had to slow down. Also the attitude of most of our colleagues at the beginning was: 'you can never organise IPE across educational programmes' while our experience is that this is not an issue at all anymore. Sometimes we were very frustrated and felt that we could not handle these barriers. However, we continued looking for opportunities, even though these were sometimes few. We had to design a multifaceted implementation of IPE to address several barriers. Some of the interventions were planned ahead and some interventions needed to be worked out, based on the ongoing developing situation.

Charismatic and participative leadership qualities of the leaders of the IP working group, focusing on low hanging fruit and small opportunities, as well as involving relevant stakeholders, especially the curriculum committees were essential. Besides, the faculty was awarded with an 'innovation grant' to develop and implement IPE two years in a row. This accelerated the development and implementation of IPE. By mouth-to-mouth stories about positive experiences of educators in IPE activities several other colleagues developed a positive attitude, became enthusiastic and joined our IP working group or as IP educators. The support of the management was and still is fundamentally together with the external urge anticipating future health care demands. This eased and still eases our work.

For anyone who has the same assignment to set up IPE might learn from our experiences and benefit from our key take home message: management support is essential, start with a sheared vision, knowledge and language, begin with adapting the already present small opportunities in the educational programmes and finally, stay patient and optimistic.

Recapitulating, setting up IPE is a challenging, time-consuming and complex task and also rewarding. For us, there is a lot to progress in the near future: further developing and implementing the IPE pathway, rigorously evaluating the IPE activities, defining and broadening the IPE community of practice, and sound faculty development activities with a sufficient reach. However, looking ahead, our prognosis is that in the academic year 2016-2017, we will be able to start the full-blown IPE pathway with all $1^{st}$ year students in all educational programmes. This means that 2019-2020 the first 'collaborative practice ready' (WHO 2010) health professionals will graduate at Zuyd. Still, a lot of boundaries need to be crossed to make our IPE road while walking.

## Acknowledgements

This chapter is written on behalf of the IP working group. The members are: Steffy Stans (occupational therapy), Jose van Oppen (physiotherapy), Thea Verstappen, (nursing), Sophie Ubben (speech & language therapy), Ronny Minnaard (biomedical technology), Ina van Keulen (arts therapy), Marieke Ploumen-Hendrix (midwifery), Sitske Horneman (social studies and education), Eva Stultiens (lifelong learning) and also Claudy Cobben-Cofcoeur (speech & language therapy), Angelique Cappa and Jolanda Friesen-Storms (nursing).

## Literature

Neville AJ (2009). Problem-based Learning and medical education forty years on. *Medical Principles and Practice*, *18*, 1–9.

Adviescommissie NLQF–EQF (2011). *Introductie van het Nederlands Nationaal Kwalificatiekader NLQF in nationaal en Europees perspectief.* 's Hertogenbosch: Commissie NLQF–EQF.

Barr H (1998). Competent to collaborate: Towards a competency-based model for interprofessional education. *Journal of Interprofessional Care*, *12*, 181-188.

Contributors in attendance at the JQI meeting in Dublin. (2004). *Shared 'Dublin' descriptors for Short Cycle, First Cycle, Second Cycle and Third Cycle Award.* Dublin: Joint Quality Initiative Informal Group.

Frank JR (2005). *The CanMEDS 2005 Physician Competency Framework. Better standards. Better physicians. Better care.* Ottawa: The Royal College of Physicians and Surgeons of Canada.

Frenk, J, Chen L, Bhutta, Z, Cohen, J, Crisp N, Evans T, Fineberg H, Garcia P, Ke Y, Kelley P, Kistnasamy B, Meleis A, Naylor D, Pablos-Mendez A, Reddy S, Scrimshaw S, Sepulveda J, Serwadda D & Zurayk H (2010). Health professionals for a new century: Transforming education to strengthen health systems in an interdependent world. *Lancet*, *376*, 1923-1958.

Garssen J (2001). *Demografie van de vergrijzing.* Den Haag / Heerlen: Centraal Buro voor de Statistiek.

Grol R & Wensing M (2004). What drives change? Barriers to and incentives for achieving a evidence-based practice. *Medical Journal*, *180*, S57-60.

Grol R, Wensing M & Eccles M (2005). *Improving patient care. The implementation of change in clinical practice.* Edinburgh: Elsevier Butterworth Heineman.

Grol R, Wensing M, Eccles M & Davis D (2013). *Improving patient care. The implementation of change in clinical practice* (2nd edition). London: Wiley Blackwell.

Mead N & Bower P (2000). Patient-centredness: A conceptual framework and review of the empirical literature. *Social Science and Medicine*, *51*, 1087-1110.

Svenaeus F (2001). *The hermeneutics of medicine and the phenomenology of health. Step towards a philosophy of medical practice.* Dordrecht: Kluwer Academic Publishers.

Vyt A (2009). *Exploring quality assurance for interprofessional education in health and social care.* Antwerpen-Apeldoorn: Garant.

World Health Organisation (2001). *International classification of functioning, disabilities and health problems.* Geneva: World Health Organisation.

WHO Working Group (2010). *Framework for action on interprofessional education and collaborative practice.* Geneva: World Health Organisation.

# IPE in undergraduate medical and health care studies: Collaboration with authorities, public services and schools

Tiina Tervaskanto-Mäentausta, Anja Taanila, Ulla-Maija Seppänen and Essi Varkki

## Local needs, health care services and education hand in hand

The health care education today is focused more on hospital care, specialized medicine and clinical skills. At the same time the period of patient care and stay in hospitals is shortening. The demand for better collaboration between specialized hospitals and outpatient care in primary health care is increasing. Personal responsibility for own health choices and lifestyle is important for everyone. More professional guidance and advice is needed to help patients. School age children and young people are the important focus groups as well as the increasing number of older people. Health care professionals need greater competence in preventing and promoting health and wellbeing.

Interprofessional education (IPE) is a necessary step in preparing a "collaborative practice-ready" health workforce (WHO 2013). Interprofessional (IP) competencies are needed for better and effective user-centred services. Collaborative practice happens when multiple health workers from different professional backgrounds work together with patients, families, carers and communities to deliver the highest quality of care. Local authorities, policy-makers and educators should plan the model of services and IP collaboration appropriate to their own local or regional context.

As stated by to the Finnish Ministry of Social Affairs and Health the aim of health care is to maintain and improve people's health, wellbeing, work and functional capacity and social security, as well as to reduce health inequalities. The Finnish health care system is based on preventive health care and well-run comprehensive health services (The MSAH 2014). These are the requirements for health care educators as well. Local needs and regional development have to be taken into account when planning the programmes and curricula. Increasing collaboration with educators and service provider partners is needed during the undergraduate studies.

Health promotion and disease prevention are the primary aims of Finnish health care policy. The National Development Plan for Social Welfare and Health Care (Kaste Programme 2015) is a strategic steering tool that is used to manage and reform social and health policy. One of the sub-programmes is to develop more effective services for children, young and families with children and another to improve services for older people (MSAH 2015). The health care needs of children, adolescents and older people have been the development themes in collaboration of the service provider partners, health and social care agencies, and the university.

Oulu University of Applied Sciences (Oulu UAS) and the University of Oulu, Faculty of Medicine (UO) have developed IPE, including common courses and training for undergraduate medical and health care students. The curriculum for health care education concerning health promotion and disease prevention skills has been developed to include IP learning (Tervaskanto-Mäentausta e.a. 2014).

The first IP course for medical and health care students in the first semester was *Public Health and Interprofessional collaboration*. The objectives of the course were that students familiarise themselves with the basis of health promotion and possibilities for interprofessional collaboration (IPC), challenges of public health, functioning of national health and social welfare systems and national strategies. Students from eight different degree programmes (physician, dentist, dental hygienist, nurse, public health nurse, midwife, paramedic, occupational therapist) have taken part in this course since 2007.

Participative learning methods including eLearning and workshops were used during the course. The eLearning part was built on family cases. The aim was that the cases would help the students to obtain a real picture of how the service system works, what kind of basic services the families can get and how the IPC of workers helps to resolve everyday problems. A student conference was the final part of the course Students prepared for the conference by writing a personal essay and an abstract in a small group. Students' attitudes to IPE and the learning experiences were evaluated annually. According to the results of the evaluation more practically-based IPE was wanted.

Common projects were the next step to develop the IP Curricula, IP Training and collaboration with service providers. In projects innovative practice-based learning environments were developed and active learning methods have been introduced. In Oulu in Finland students from several degree programmes have participated in the projects as trainers, developers and researchers during their undergraduate studies. The Lancet Commission (2013) recommends using blended learning in IPE. Several studies have demonstrated an overall positive effect of e-learning or blended learning courses compared to the more traditional didactic teaching in the acquisition and retention of knowledge.

# Interprofessional training in primary and specialized care

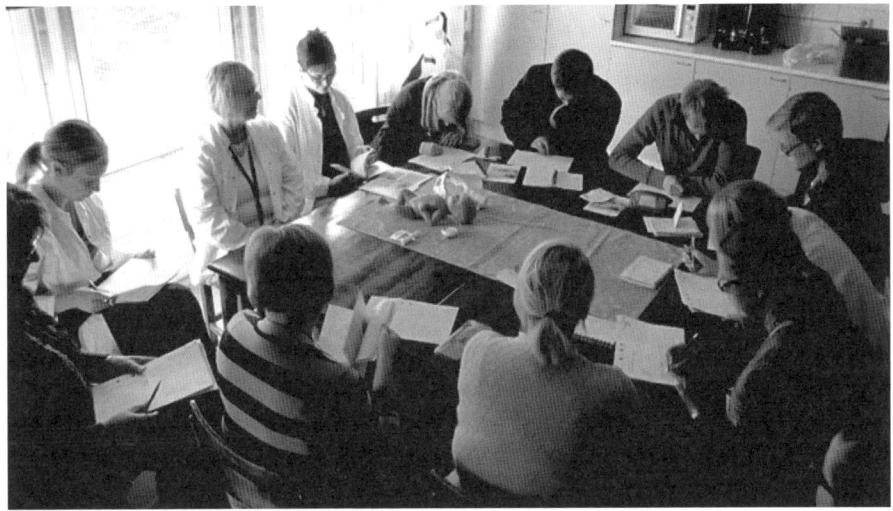

The INNOPI (ESF) project (2008-2012) aimed to develop innovative learning environments for IP learning. The partners in the project came both from the Universities of Oulu and from their most important service providers from the City of Oulu and from Oulu University Hospital.

## Interprofessional training in maternity and child health care clinics.

One subproject was to pilot IP training in maternity and child health care clinics. IP pair training periods were implemented in collaboration with the Oulu primary health care centre, with UO and with Oulu UAS. Fifth-year medical students (n=101) and fourth year public health nurses (n=31) and teachers participated in the training programme during 2010-2012. The study aimed to investigate students' attitudes and readiness for interprofessional learning (IPL), and at strengthening their professional skills and at gathering clients' experiences. The second aim was to strengthen students' professional skills by working with clients using a client-centred approach. The third aim was to gather and evaluate clients' experiences after the clinical visit (Tervaskanto-Mäentausta e.a. 2014).

Students were divided in IP pairs. Facilitators were named for each pair. The pairs planned the procedure of the visit, and examined the client. In addition, they observed and reflected the work of the others. A tool for observers was modified from Anaesthetists' Non-technical Skills (ANTS, 2012). It consisted of several areas including task management, teamwork, situation awareness, patient-centredness, and professional decision making. One pair took care of the client's visit independently, while another pair observed their working. Then the roles of the student pairs were switched so that finally all pairs completed all the tasks. All together six clients were examined during one day. Facilitators, doctors and nurses, were at all times available to guide and help where needed. The feedback was collected from all the students (response rate 100%) and the clients (n=94) by using questionnaires.

The results showed that the training promoted pair work skills of the students (Figure 15). IPL was considered important during the pair training. The students considered that they learned preventive and holistic patient and family centred care. Positive experiences promoted learning but some of the students felt that they did not have enough earlier experience to fully benefit from this type of training and that they had not been prepared well enough. The professional roles of both professions were better understood and the students learned how to support each other. Overall the students had become familiar with the preventive health care system during the training session (Tervaskanto-Mäentausta e.a. 2014). Their comments were positive:

> "I had good experiences of how the public health nurse and the doctor can support each other's work".

> "Collaboration with the nurse student guided me to think from a different point of view".

> "It was challenging to work in a team and in the same time to keep the focus in the patient during the visit".

> "It was important to remember to support the parents and the family".

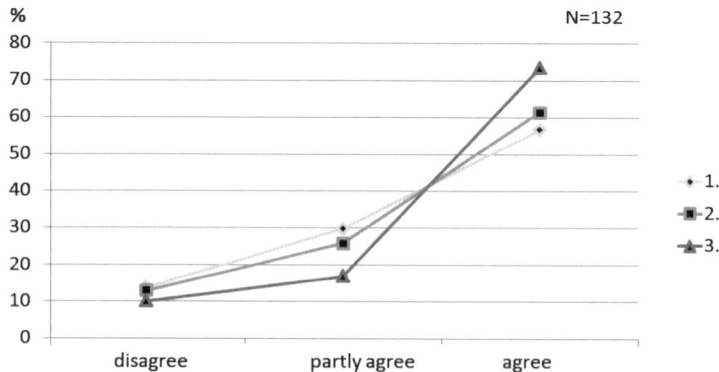

Figure 15: Evaluation of the impact of pair work on three aspects: promotion of pair work skills (1), understanding the importance of collaboration (2), and clarification of the view of preventive and holistic health care (3).

## Interprofessional care of diabetes patients in the health care centre

Improving primary services and facilitating early interventions in public health problems are pivotal challenges according to the Finnish National Development Programme for Social Welfare and Health Care (Kaste 2012-15). Oulu UAS and UO planned and organised IP pilots together with the Oulu Health Care Centre. Groups of two medical students and one nursing student planned and carried out an outpatient visit to primary health care patients with diabetes and obesity. These patients were chosen since diabetes and obesity are among the most important public health issues in developed countries today.

The aims of the study were to investigate students' attitudes towards IP training and learning. Teachers from both the universities, a doctor and a diabetes nurse from the health care centre planned and organised the pilots. The students were third-year medical and fourth-year nurse students. The patients were diabetes type 2 (DM2) patients or obese DM2 patients. A group had to take care of one patient visit independently. Material was prepared for the students, such as recommendations of the evidence base for care and guidelines for patient examination. After this general information all participating students became familiar with the patients' prior medical history together with the facilitating doctor and nurse. Altogether 69 students and 23 patients participated in the pilots 2012-2014.

Students' attitudes towards IPE were evaluated with RIPLS (Readiness for Interprofessional Learning Scale) (Parsell & Bligh 1999). They agreed strongly that trusting each other is important when working in a team. Students felt that it was important to learn to work together during the undergraduate studies in order to become a good team worker in the future. They agreed strongly that the patients benefit most from the fact that professionals work as a team. Clinical skills as well as communicational skills were learned. In respect of roles and responsibilities one half of the students thought that nurses and doctors have their own skills and tasks. Half also thought that they have to learn more than the other professionals. When evaluating the learning, students felt they still have to learn much more how to use all information about the patient's holistic situation, other diseases, strengths and resources for good care (Figure 16).

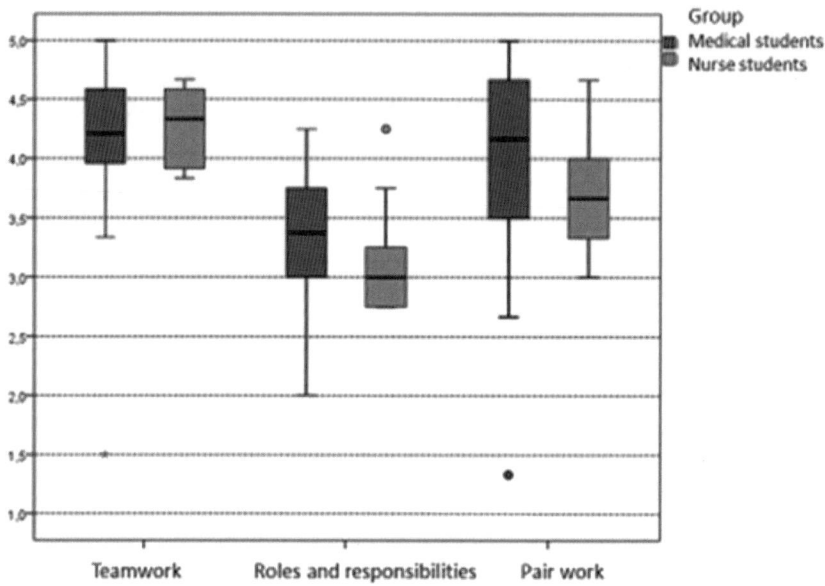

Figure 16: Students attitudes and readiness towards IPL.

Students perceived they had adequate skills in teamwork, creating a trusting atmosphere, using good questions to find out the problems of patients, treating them with respect and noticing nonverbal communication. These pilots have provided valuable models for further organising and developing IP training in the primary health care sector, which is increasingly responsible for patients with chronic and long-term illnesses. The role of a nurse has become more independent, as they now often work as a pair with the doctor. Improved collaboration between specialized hospital care and outpatient care in the primary setting are also required.

### Interprofessional training environment in a hospital ward

The first pilot of the training ward model was implemented in the respiratory ward of Oulu University hospital in April 2011 after careful planning and sustained collaboration between the Medical Faculty of UO, Oulu UAS and staff from Oulu University Hospital. The Swedish model from Linköping (Wilhelmsson e.a. 2009) was used as a guide, but local health needs and local curricula of both Universities were taken into consideration from the very beginning. Medical and nursing students also gave their input in planning the week.

In the first pilot two medical students and two nursing students worked in medical-nursing student pairs taking care of respiratory patients as a part of IP team for the period of one week. The students worked under the supervision and guidance of a respiratory nurse and a respiratory physician. The pilot received very positive feedback from the students, teachers, respiratory ward staff and patients, and the training ward model was therefore decided to be continued and developed further. Since the first pilot in 2011, more professions, physiotherapy and recently pharmacy, have been added to the student team. In addition to the respiratory ward, IP clinical practice has now been conducted on the cardiology ward and the model has been implemented in the internal medicine ward of district hospital of Kokkola. In addition there are opportunities for new IP training pilots from the surgical ward (urology) and gynaecology.

The aim of implementing the training ward model was to improve teaching, learning and clinical practice within IP team. The aim of the IP clinical practice has been to familiarize students from different professions with working together, to learn about each other and to learn from each other during their studies. An additional aim has been to improve students' teamwork, interaction and co-operation skills, and to enhance learning, understanding and valuing each other's expertise.

Students have been generally very satisfied with IP clinical practice. According to their evaluation forms students felt they had learned about each other's professional duties. Not only students, but teachers too felt they had learnt from each other. All patients participating in different pilots felt they received a good quality of care from the students. Teachers and student facilitators were convinced that the IP clinical practice week provided abundantly meaningful learning opportunities for all students and that IP clinical practice is an effective way to learn about different professionals. It enhances teamwork and helps students to grow into their own professional roles.

From the beginning of planning these pilots, it has been noted on several occasions that implementation of successful IPE requires careful planning and determined and sustained collaboration between IPE faculties and the local health care provider. In the future we aim to establish our very own IP training ward implemented in the curricula and available to all students at some point in their studies.

## Interprofessional training with children and adolescents

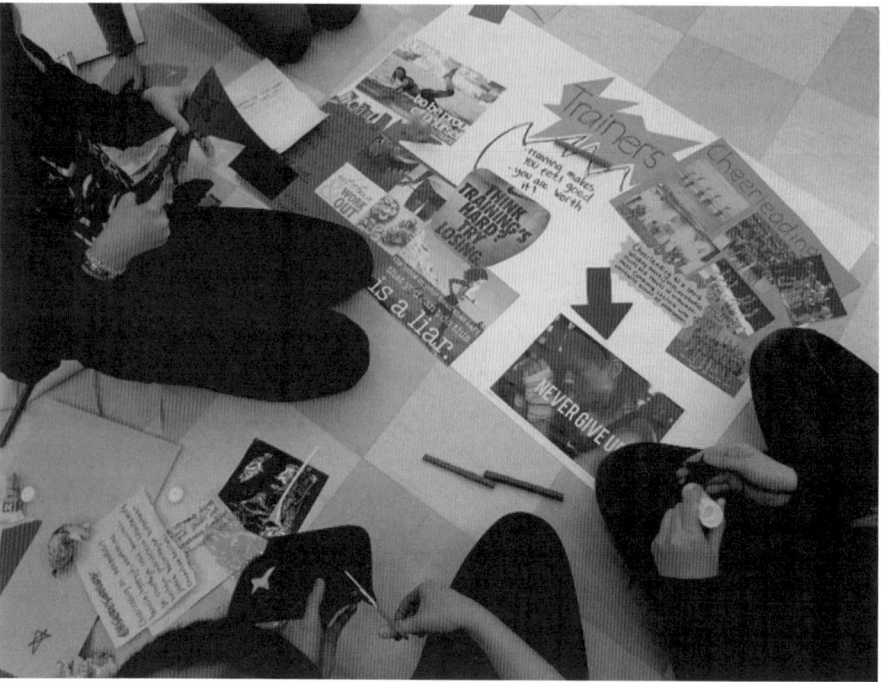

For several years Oulu UAS has collaborated with primary and secondary schools concerning health and wellbeing promotion for school age children. Two teachers are members of the national network *School Health Ambassadors*. The network is connected to the National Institute for Health and Welfare of Finland, which is responsible for organising the biennial School Health Promotion (SHP) study. The SHP monitors the health and well-being of Finnish 14–20-year-old adolescents. The aim of the SHP study is to strengthen the planning and evaluation of health promotion activities at school and at municipal and national levels. The study includes 84% of the age group in comprehensive schools and 70% in upper secondary schools. The study provides an opportunity to monitor trends and assess differences between genders and areas. In school settings, the results can be utilized in the planning and evaluating of health education and co-operation between different professionals and students (SHP 2014).

*Hello Future!* is an action model developed in the city of Oulu to promote authorities and parents working together for the healthier future of school-aged children and adolescents. It utilizes the SHP results. The main aims of the model are to strengthen youth participation and to cooperate with families, officials and other authorities with the same goal. Oulu UAS students, from Finland or other countries and on several different degree programmes (nursing, physiotherapy, occupational therapy, midwifery, and social care), have organised health and wellbeing projects in collaboration with secondary schools in Oulu every year since 2008.

The pedagogical aim of these projects has been to develop a pupil-centred approach to learning and understanding ones' emotions on health and wellbeing choices for life and future. The aim for the students is to learn prevention and health promotion in an innovative and inspiring way while working in an IP group. The students make a project plan, in which the results of the SHP for the school provide the research basis of the project, including risks and strengths. The results of the SHP are not shared with the pupils as such, but used during the process when working together, since pupils are asked to define those themes they find most important for their own health and wellbeing in the future. After the important issues have been identified, the pupils continue working in small groups. The student's role is to be the group leader. During the process the groups prepare a product (film, game etc.) or message to the adults (poster or PowerPoint-presentation) of the issue as they have defined it.

This type of project has been a new method for the university students to study and learn. Session by session students learn more about the pupils and their thinking, about working with students from different professions, about different methods and most of all about their own attitudes and skills for health promotion and prevention. To organise studies like this is challenging for the teachers as well. The teachers' role is different. It includes negotiation with schools beforehand as well as briefing the students to make the project plan and facilitating the implementation of the project and evaluating learning.

According to student feedback, they have never had such strong IP work experience during their previous studies. They evaluated the work as challenging, but the results had been successful and satisfying. They learned to look at health and wellbeing in a different way and also how to teach and supervise teenaged pupils with health issues in an interesting way. This method of studying is preparing students for the 21st century skills (Dede 2009). According to their feedback the students have learned more skills for inventive thinking, effective communication, personal and social responsibility, creativity and innovation as well as critical thinking, problem solving and decision making. Both the students and the school where pupils are studying have gathered feedback from the pupils. Their opinion is that this project is one of the highlights of their eight year studies.

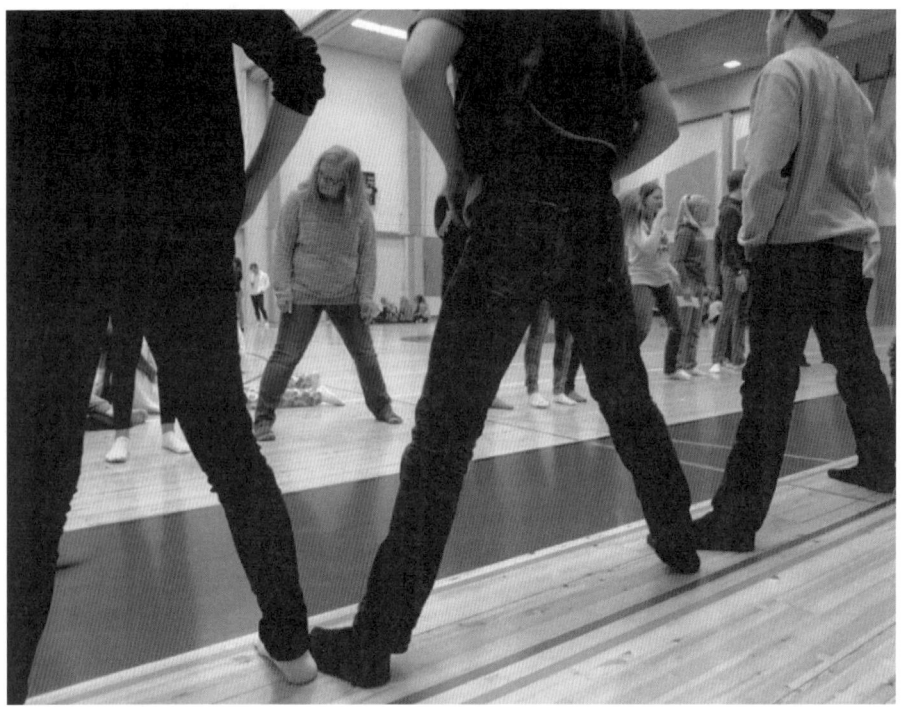

In the City of Oulu voluntary high school tutors are trained in cooperation with Oulu UAS since 2010. High school counsellors and teachers from Oulu UAS organise the training together. Oulu UAS' students carry out two parts of that education programme as a part of their professional studies: understanding the group process and the power of a group when working as a tutor.

Oulu UAS' students and international exchange students from different degree programmes (nurse, public health nurse, physiotherapist, occupational therapist, midwife, social care), plan and implement the tutor training project. The aim is to train high school students to become tutors for new high school students in the next semester. Peer tutors have an important role promoting the health and wellbeing of their school mates. Every spring about 150 students from 11 high schools participate in the training project. The aim of the training is that the high school students learn the skills and methods of being a tutor in order to support the wellbeing of others. A tutor's role is to guide and support other high school students in any situations where help and guidance are needed and to understand the principles of healthy life style choices.

The tasks for the university students are to plan, carry out and evaluate the project for health and wellbeing promotion. A Facebook group has been the usual platform for IP working and collaboration during the project.

The project consists of two parts. The aim of the first part is grouping: getting to know each other, to trust and to resolve problematic situations with which tutor students may be faced. This task enhances the tutor students' knowledge about the different methods they can use when tutoring their new school mates in situations they may face in real school life. The tutor students are divided into four groups and each session takes three hours. The second part of the project is a health and wellbeing day, organised in "stations" and topics. The topics are chosen according to the results of the SHP.

Participants' evaluation data have been collected after each grouping session and after the health and wellbeing day. According to the feedback, this was the first time during their studies that they had experienced such strong IP work experience. The tutors gained skills and tools. They were trained to resolve problematic situations and to talk about difficult issues. In general the project was evaluated as successful and positive. University students provided evaluations of their learning as well. They learned about project work and working with the adolescents. They learned to work as an IP team and to share responsibilities. They also learned about different health and social professions, health promotion and cultures.

## Developing services for older people in joint projects

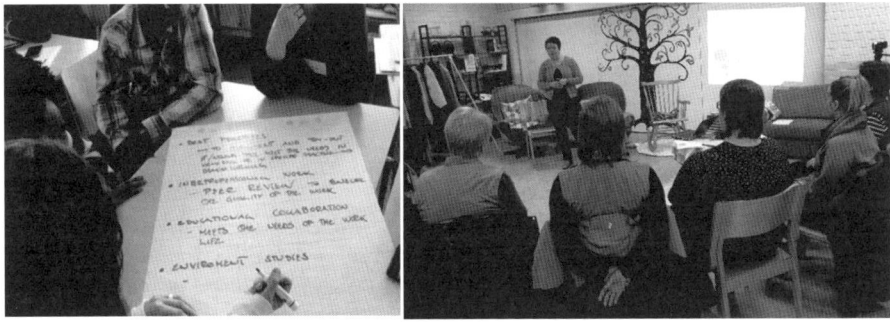

The purpose of the *Harmonious twilight of my life–project* 2011-2014 funded by the European Social Fund (ESF) was to create service models which improve the independent managing and health of the ageing population. It includes client/patient-centred qualitative care, IP collaboration, interdisciplinary under- and postgraduate education as well as research and the development of innovations. Partners of the project included Oulu UAS and the UO, the private and public senior housing organisations from Oulu region and international partners from Denmark and Italy. The objectives of the project were to compare national and international experiences in the quality of daily living and customer processes for elderly people, produce innovative ways to organise services for the elderly people and organise education for the workers and professionals in these services.

Under- and post-graduate students from Oulu UAS were recruited to the project as developers and researchers as a part of their studies and for their final theses. They trained and worked in the municipality and in the senior houses together with elderly people, their relatives and their carers. At the same time the teachers as project workers collaborated with the stakeholders and international partners.

All the partners had their own tasks. In the community and in senior houses the goal was to strengthen collaboration with the elderly, their relatives and the staff to mobilise and energise the residents and to recognize the changes in functional ability early enough. Other tasks included improving the integration process between community and senior houses and to strengthen the community of the elderly people. The task for the professionals and students was to increase their knowledge about elderly care and their IP teamwork skills.

In spring 2014 an international workshop was organised to share best practices in elderly care, to improve IP team work and to plan educational collaboration . New ideas for better care of the elderly were brainstormed. It was decided to continue with sharing best practices, continuing educational collaboration between the educators and service providers/partners and networking towards better elderly care.

Twenty seven students wrote their final theses during the project (Figure 17). These papers are now data for a doctoral thesis. The focus is now to develop a process for selecting the best ideas for development of innovations from users' needs and grass root level practice (Thomas e.a. 2005).

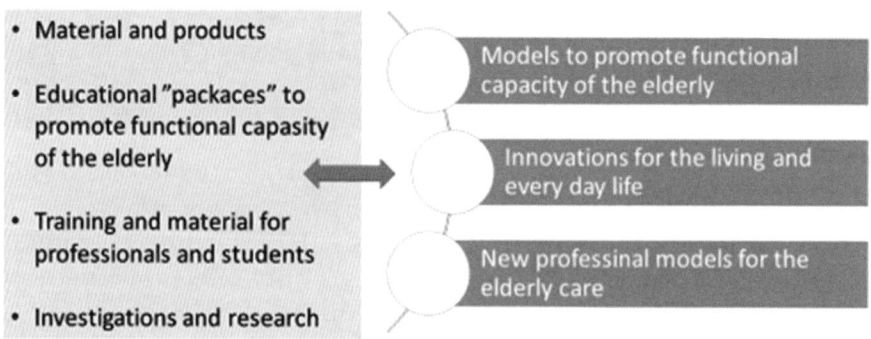

Figure 17: Final thesis of the students based on project aims.

## Focus for the future and for new innovations

The City of Oulu set up a working group to plan an IPL environment for medical, health and social care students. Participants were from the regional higher education institutes and vocational schools and the city of Oulu and Oulu University hospital. The goal was to create an IP training environment in the new Kontinkangas wellbeing centre. All health and wellbeing services were planned to be under the same roof. The idea was to make these services flexible for the users. Working in the IP teams aims to improve better and effective care of the clients.

The CAMPUS 2014–project (ESF) aimed to increase IP and pedagogical skills of teachers and staff to supervise IP student teams training in primary health care facilities. Partners in the project were Oulu UAS, UO, Oulu Vocational College, Diaconia University of Applied Sciences and City of Oulu. The CAMPUS project organised two sets of training courses for teachers and professionals; these focused on IPE and facilitating the IP students' teams. The aim of the training courses was to innovate and develop IP models for training with different focus groups in the new wellbeing centre. The course plan was based on the national strategy towards user-centred care and service (Figure 18).

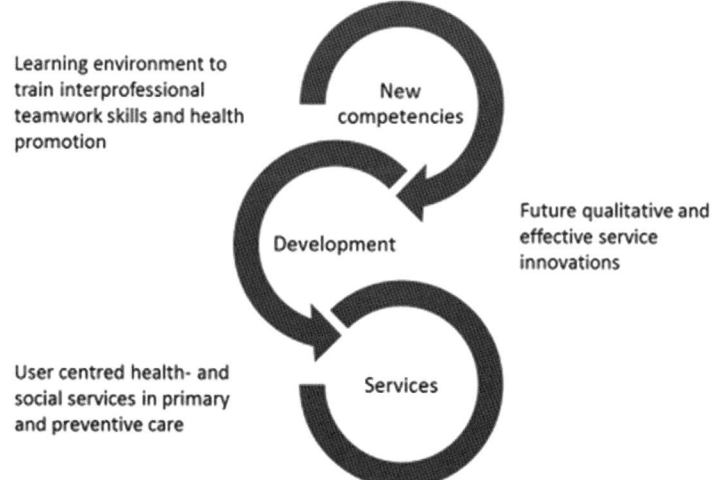

Figure 18: Focus areas of the CAMPUS project.

The Kontinkangas IP wellbeing centre was opened in January 2015. In collaboration with the city of Oulu and the educational organisations IP training practices continued and developed further. There are challenges in finding suitable facilities and mutual times for training, but positive learning experiences of students and feedback from service users encourage continuation.

IP health and social care education has taken a huge leap forward in the Oulu area. The next step will be to expand the network. The Kontinkangas campus area in Oulu provides possibilities for close collaboration with the educational and health and social service organisations, since all institutions are located within walking distance from each other. All those organisations together with the health and wellbeing technology companies compose the Oulu Health ecosystem. Oulu Health is linked to the European Connected Health Alliance (see www.echalliance.com/ecosystems/).

ECHAlliance Ecosystems bring together communities connecting health, wellbeing and social care stakeholders interested in developing a joint health agenda across a specific country or region. The target of the Ecosystems is to strengthen partnerships and to expedite the adoption of solutions to challenges in health and social care (Figure 19). All stakeholders benefit from collaboration.

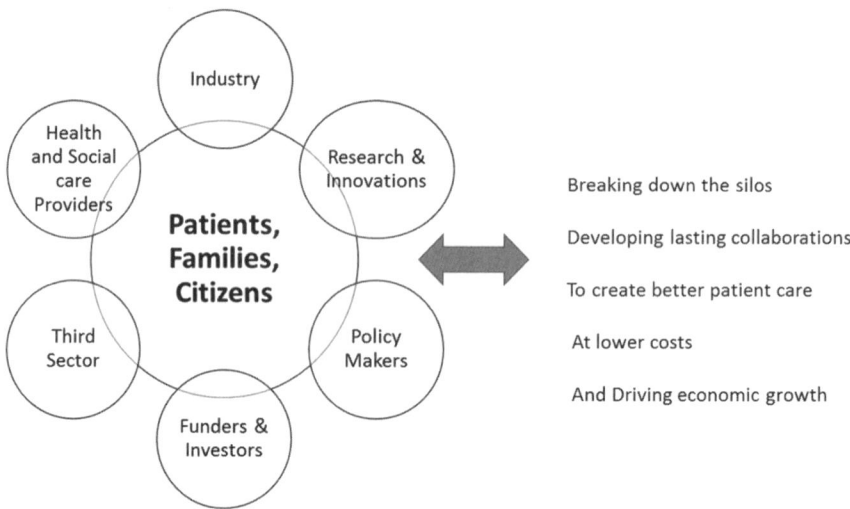

Figure 19: Structure of health and social care ecosystem.

The health and wellbeing sector is in a process of technological revolution. New innovations are needed, for example in facing the challenges of a demographic transition. New approaches are needed for example when the population is getting older. More and more ICT innovations and mobile applications have been created to personalize health care. An ongoing challenge for companies in the health and welfare sectors, is the lack of infrastructure that would support health, welfare and medical technology development in collaboration between public and private agents. On the other hand, health care professionals are in a need of suitable platforms and partner networks to enable implementation of their work-related innovations.

Oulu Labs (ERF) is the newest project coordinating by Oulu university hospital in partnership with city of Oulu and Oulu UAS. Oulu Health Labs project will develop a systematic approach to enable and support the development of health and medical technology products and services in a user-oriented way. The goal is to provide productized development, innovation and a testing platform to support new product market entries and utilization of innovative solutions. The project is built on unique collaboration between project partners, companies, research and educational institutes and health care service users within Oulu Health ecosystem. The Oulu Sote Labs project will establish functions, including:

- Test lab facilities
- Technology Health Care Center Oulu– testing and analyzing services in real healthcare environment
- Structured collaboration method between health care professionals and companies
- Interprofessional innovation workshops and rapid prototyping
- Collaboration projects with Nordic test beds

To conclude, future medical, health and social care education will have plenty of opportunities to carry out IPE. Collaboration and networking, as well as integrating education in existing working life networks and development projects, will provide students with the competencies needed in their future professional practice.

## Literature

ANTS (2012). Anaesthetists' Non-Technical Skills (ANTS): System Handbook v1.0. University of Aberdeen.

Dede C (2009). Comparing Frameworks for "21st Century Skills". Available at http://www.p21.orhttp://citeseerx.ist.psu.edu/viewdoc/download?doi=10.1.1.475.3846&rep=rep1&type=pdfg/storage/documents/P21_Framework_Definitions.pdf

KASTE Programme (2015). National Development Programme for Social Welfare and Health Care (Kaste). Available at http://stm.fi/en/kaste-progamme

The Lancet Commission (2010). Health professionals for a new century: Transforming education to strengthen health systems in an interdependent world. *Lancet, 376*, 1923–1958.

MSAH (2015). The Finnish Ministry of Social Affairs and Health: Welfare and health promotion. http://stm.fi/en/promotion-of-welfare

Parsell G & Bligh J (1999). The development of a questionnaire to assess the readiness of health care students for interprofessional learning (RIPLS). *Medical Education, 33*, 95-100.

SHP (2015). The School Health Promotion (SHP) study. National Institute for Health and Welfare.

Tervaskanto-Mäentausta T, Ojaniemi M, Mikkilä L, Laitila-Özcok L, Niinimäki M, Nordström T & Taanila A (2014). Collaborative learning in Maternity and Child Health Clinics. *Creative Education, 5*, 1804-1811.

Thomas P, McDonnell J, McCulloch J, White A, Bosanquet N & Ferlie E (2005). Increasing capacity for innovation in bureaucratic Primary Care organizations: A Whole System Participatory Action Research Project 2005. *Annals of Family Medicine, 3*, 312-317.

WHO (2010). Framework for Action on Interprofessional Education & Collaborative Practice. WHO/HRH/HPN/10.3

# Focused interprofessional courses: Aiming for effective competence acquisition

Andre Vyt and Bianka Vandaele

## The InterDis project and course unit in Ghent

Artevelde University College has the longest history of IPE in Belgium. The first experiments with interprofessional learning date back to the early 1990s, first by organising small-group discussion sessions in which students from different study programmes explained their profession on the basis of clinical cases. Over the next few years, IPE developed from single sessions into a series of teaching and learning activities, called the InterDis elective trajectory. In 2001 the Artevelde University College received an innovation grant from the Flemish government, to develop it further in collaboration with the Faculty of Medicine and Health Sciences at the University of Ghent. Since 2007 InterDis has been implemented as a mandatory course of 3 ECTS credits in several study programmes at the Artevelde University College (occupational therapy, speech therapy, audiology, podiatry) and in the physiotherapy programme of the University of Ghent. It has also been implemented in some measure in other departments (medicine, nursing, midwifery, dietetics, and psychology). Each year more than 600 students enrol in the course.

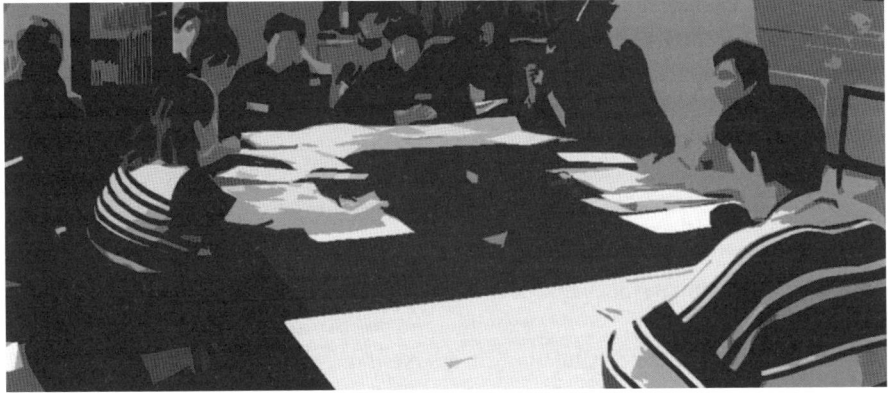

Students discussing a patient situation from different perspectives in a session of InterDis.

A clear difference with other initiatives in the region is that the InterDis course spans over more than three months, giving opportunity for students to develop their IP competences alongside other courses and with clinical practice. The trajectory includes a preparatory stage within the students' own discipline before participating in four interprofessional half-day team sessions with 12 to 15 participants. In these IP sessions they collaborate intensively with at least four other disciplines in simulated team meetings, discussing real-life situations and planning shared care for a series of patient cases. Each team is supervised by a team coach in the team sessions, while students are also supervised by a coach from their own study programme. The team coach focuses on the development and evaluation of IP competences for each team member while the other coaches are responsible for the preparation of the participating students from their own discipline and for the supplementary assignments. This complementary coaching formula allows an assessment from two separate points of view. The programme-based coaches can provide additional information about students in case the team coach needs this.

In the InterDis course unit the following five key competences have been defined:

- Consult and collaborate effectively in IP teams, on the basis of knowledge of competences of health care workers
- Develop patient-centred shared care plans on the basis of information and interaction with other health care workers
- Anticipate, identify, and remediate problems in interprofessional teamwork and shared care planning
- Make appropriate referrals to other health care workers based on the knowledge of competences of health care workers
- Evaluate interprofessional communication, decision making and care planning in terms of adequacy, effectiveness and efficiency

Five handling dimensions were identified applicable to several competences:

- Consult and collaborate
- Involve and stimulate colleagues
- Communicate and inform
- Learn and reflect
- Act and advise

Each of the five dimensions have been broken down into performance criteria linked to one or more competences. For example, the performance criteria for 'consult and collaborate' include the formulation of intervention goals in such a way that they can be integrated in a shared care plan, working constructively with others in formulating shared care goals, and selecting relevant clinical data in view of shared care planning.

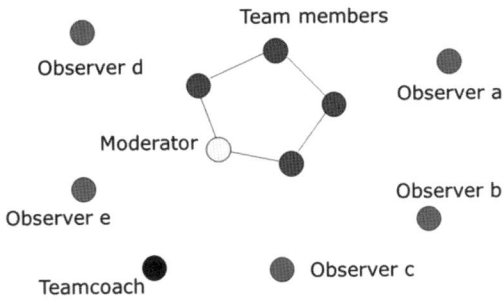

Figure 20: layout of a typical interprofessional team meeting simulation in the InterDis course unit, with 5 active team members in the middle, of which one leads the discussion as a moderator, surrounded by 5 observers and a teamcoach.

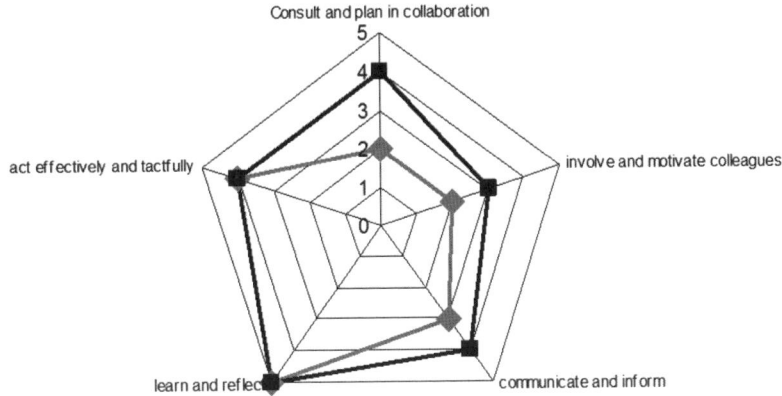

Figure 21: A profile of the five handling dimensions of two students. Both of them score very high on learning and reflecting, but one of them scores poorly on the actual consulting and planning in collaboration, involving colleagues of other professions.

The InterDis trajectory aims to ensure a competence-based assessment for each participating student. Each student has two occasions of taking a role as an active participant in a simulated team meeting, and receives focused feedback from the coach and from colleagues on his/her behavioural performance. If the student fails to demonstrate sufficient competence they will have further opportunity to show improved performance on the basis of feedback received from the coach. For this, 30 specific behavioural criteria have been defined in the form of a checklist, and a reduced set of 10 key criteria are used for assessment of critical aspects. If students do not meet each of these 10 criteria or have not acquired the five key competences, they will not pass the course or earn the credits.

As well as receiving direct feedback from the coaches, students have to perform self-assessments based on feedback received from their peers. Students observe each other based on the criteria, and reflect on the quality of individuals' behaviour as well as on team performance and the shared care planning processes and products. At the end of the trajectory, each student receives a narrative written feedback with a description of the strong and remaining weak points. In this evaluation the coaches include the student's preparatory activities and the performance on additional assignments (reflective papers, minutes of meetings, detailed shared care plans, and thematic report papers). A portfolio system combined with behavioural scoring provides a full evaluation of the interprofessional competence of the student.

Students whose performance appears not to meet the IP competences are discussed in a staff meeting with coaches, as a double check to ensure the same evaluation standards have been applied to all students. Since the InterDis course unit is very much competence-focused with clear assessment criteria and processes, and final-year students are intensively coached, the pass rate is very high. The percentage of failures is usually less than 2%. Cross-checking with performance on other course units makes clear that failing students usually also have a problem with their performance in clinical practice. This finding corroborates the validity of the method used in InterDis. While the sessions remain at the level of simulation, and patients do not participate, assessment focuses on behaviour related to clinical practice. Students are required to assume their role as realistically as possible.

The student guide informs students at the start of the course about the learning objectives and the working methods, and also the roles and responsibilities of the coaches. It is necessary for the student to have clinical experience before or during the course, since practice-based reflection is an essential element in the learning process. An initial self-assessment is the very important starting point. Students assess for themselves whether they have the required entry competences to assure that they have a good foundation for the learning trajectory. A cross-check with their actual performance is completed in the first session. Sometimes this can be very at variance with their self-assessment.

The entry skills or competences that are required to enrol in the course, are:

- Listen actively and consult/confer in a small group
- Formulate his/her own opinion in a clear and differentiated way
- Report (in written) an action or a consultation
- Evaluate intervention possibilities of from the own profession
- Write up a diagnostic profile based on the ICF-framework
- Write up a plan for intervention and care from the own profession
- Formulate working goals, and adjust these on the basis of feedback

If students lack any required knowledge or skills at entry, they are required to remediate this in the preparatory phase with the help of the coach from their own programme. This procedure has been introduced to ensure that team functioning is not hindered by the few students who fail on prerequisites. Since the trajectory comprises a limited number of team sessions, the working formula is aimed at efficiency in coaching. Coaches identify students who fail on behavioural performance and provide them with additional feedback and opportunity to learn. Students with a high level of behavioural performance may be given the opportunity to act as a moderator in a session, or to assist the coach in the discussion on reflection with the students based on their observations. At the end of the trajectory, students provide feedback about the quality of the preparation, coaching, and assessment.

Specific attention is applied to the use of ICF. We have experienced that, while students generally have already learned to use this model actively in clinical reasoning, they frequently do this from a profession specific viewpoint, and not always consider the patient's context and needs at the forefront. For example, physiotherapy students frequently learn to reason from the physiological level to the activity level and then move to the implications on the level of social participation. The patients' needs, strengths and weaknesses, but also the contextual elements are added frequently as an annex or an additional point of attention.

In the InterDis sessions, students learn to change the direction of reasoning together with reframing the goalsetting. Instead of focusing on profession-specific goals and putting these together in care planning, they learn to start with defining interprofessional goals on the basis of patients' specifics. They learn to reason as a health care worker from the perspective of the patient instead of as a specific professional on the basis of professional skills. For a number of students this requires a major shift in reasoning. The course acts as an eye-opener in terms of the role of a health care team member.

A second important tool is the shared care matrix (Vyt 2008 2012). In applying this matrix students learn to assume joint responsibilities for interprofessional care goals, and identify which of the health care workers may best monitor this goal or coordinate care to achieve the goal. This may be dependent on a concrete situation and is not necessarily linked to the specific competences of a profession. A nurse can, for example, have a very important role in assisting the monitoring of speech and hearing progress when visiting the patient daily. Students learn also to actively support each other instead of defending their own professional boundaries. For example, an occupational therapist, a physiotherapist and a nurse can jointly contribute to improve the mobility of a patient for the execution of activities of daily life.

Two collaborating coordinators are responsible for the organisation of the learning trajectory, including quality assurance and continuous quality improvement. The course team consists of 20 to 25 staff members who act as team coaches. A guide for coaches contains specific guidelines for coaching and assessment. New coaches receive training based on videotaped sessions with experienced coaches. They also have the opportunity to act as an assistant coach for one year before actively taking on the role of coach. Every year a workshop for coaches is organised around a special theme. Staff competence is also ensured by the setting of minimal requirements in experience with group learning and collaborative work. This ensures maximal coaching support on the basis of authentic experience.

Students are asked to bring their experience from clinical placements into discussions during the preparatory meetings, the IP team meetings, or the reflective meetings. On these occasions it is important that a coach can moderate discussions based on his/her own experience. The personal sharing of experience is seen as an important pillar in the teaching and learning process. Students have also to participate at least once in a multiprofessional meeting in clinical practice during their trajectory, on which they have to provide a report based on a structured evaluation. A rule of thumb is that, as early as possible, each student must receive feedback on competence aspects to be improved. For this reason small group learning was selected as the leading teaching method on InterDis.

Institutions may still avoid establishing an IP course on the argument that IP competences are already integrated in the learning outcomes of different course units and a separate IP course would lead to overlap or duplication. The embedding of IP competences in the whole curriculum is certainly an asset, providing opportunities for the gradual acquisition of competences and preventing the perception of interprofessional collaboration as an isolated or singular event. But on the other hand, it is necessary to have a clearly identifiable assessment of the IP competences, ensuring that students acquire them effectively. A specific course in which students are assessed explicitly on IP competences is a good way to ensure this.

## The IPCHC project and course unit in Antwerp

The pioneering project at the University of Ghent in the 1990s inspired other institutions in Belgium and the Netherlands after the turn of the century. The project *Interprofessional Collaboration in Health Care* (IPCHC) was organised for the first time in the Antwerp Higher Education area in the academic year 2004-2005. This project includes students from the Faculty of Medicine and Health Sciences (University of Antwerp) and from the departments of health, social care and dietetics at the Artesis Plantijn University College and Karel-de-Grote University College, and from the department of psychology and speech therapy at the Thomas

Moore University College. Recently there has also been a collaboration with Hogeschool Zeeland in the Netherlands.

The competences for a member of an interprofessional team ('Interprofessional collaborator') were developed based on the basic competences of a health care provider as formulated in the CanMeds 2000 project. The learning outcomes are based on the roles of an Interprofessional collaborator in health care: Communicator, Health Advocate, Teamplayer, Manager, Professional, Scholar and Expert. An emphasis is laid on the use of specific professional and communicative skills, and an open attitude towards the contribution of other professionals in health care.

The IPCHC project is a one-week module. All final-year students from the different departments learn to work together in an interprofessional context. Students are allocated to learning groups of twelve students from a variety of study programmes. Each group of 12 to 14 students is guided by a trained tutor. The task of the tutor is to guide, observe and evaluate the group and the individuals on their progress and performance during the week. The project includes lectures, self-directed learning, group work, reflection and feedback. Students learn to debate efficiently and effectively to resolve patient cases and interdisciplinary care situations. The module ends with a plenary session and discussion, where students are confronted with experts' personal experience of interprofessional care as a patient or professional. In order to appreciate the level to which students have already developed some skills or competence levels as an interprofessional collaborator, they are evaluated by self- and peer assessment and the construction of a personal portfolio.

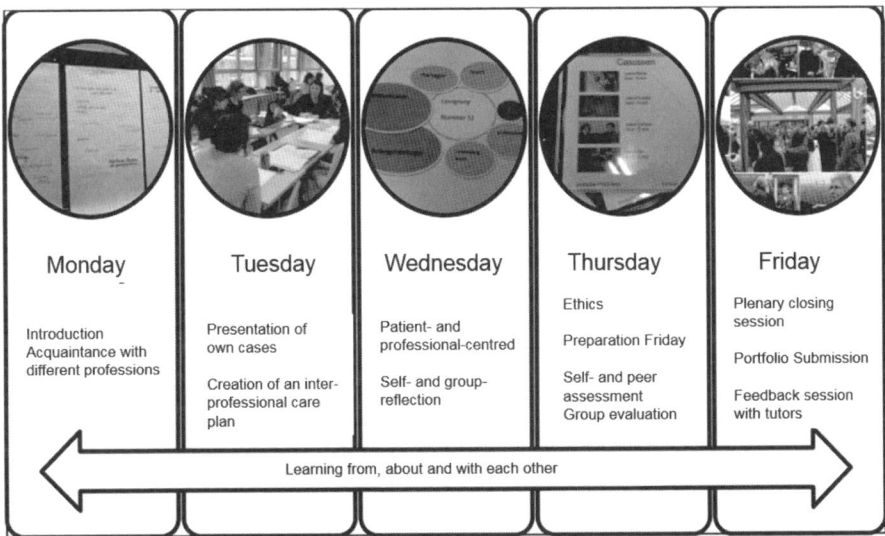

Figure 20: Course layout of the interprofessional week in Antwerp.

One of the main success factors of this project has been the multidisciplinary steering group in which subteams have taken responsibility for organisational and logistical aspects as well as for programme development. Each study programme has a representative on the steering group. These people then inform their head of department, students and colleagues.

Since 2010 an interprofessional training module has been available for health professionals in educational practice. This consists of an introductory session and three consultancy sessions. The participating health professionals (medical specialists, general practitioners, physiotherapists, nurses, social workers and occupational therapists) are divided into small interdisciplinary groups, guided by one tutor. They have three meetings where participants introduce and discuss their case studies, i.e. work situations where they have experienced problems in interprofessional collaboration. They describe the context, what happened, and how they were involved. The group participants interact and learn through reflection, looking for a deeper understanding of the context, interpersonal relationships and alternative approaches to communication and collaboration.

## Undergraduate and postgraduate programmes

It already is a good thing if undergraduate programmes in health and social care incorporate course units or modules that focus on interprofessional collaboration. An effective acquisition of a range of interprofessional competences however requires a re-engineering or a shift in the global organisation and the content of a study programme. Also, postgraduate programmes can be developed for specific target groups in which interprofessional collaboration is crucial. This is, for example, the case for the programme *Interprofessional care for older persons*, started recently at the PXL University College in Hasselt. Throughout a period of one or two years, students already working as a professional develop projects and collaborate on assignments based on their own experience and adjusted to their specific work context.

Bringing health professionals from a similar setting together, working with similar target groups but from a variety of professional backgrounds is an ideal situation to achieve a real change in the competence profile and in the daily work routine of professionals. It allows participants to learn in a way that allows the individuals' transfer of interprofessional learning to their practice setting and their changed professional practice. They can be motivated to help to develop wider changes in the organisation and delivery of care (Table 8). Implementing IP course units in undergraduate studies delivers cohorts of qualified professionals, but this is insufficient to bring about the change needed in accordance with the latest WHO reports (WHO 2010 2015).

Table 8: Modified version of Kirkpatrick's (1967) outcomes model, as modified by Barr et al. (2000, see also Hammick et al., 2007). Additionally the level of behavioural change could be divided in a level comprising the acquisition of a competence in simulated conditions (3a) and in real practice (3b).

| | |
|---|---|
| 1. Reaction | Learners' views on the learning experience and its interprofessional nature |
| 2a. Modification of perceptions and attitudes | Changes in reciprocal attitudes or perceptions between participant groups; changes in perception or attitudes towards the value and/or use of team approaches to caring for a specific client group |
| 2b. Acquisition of knowledge and skills | Including knowledge and skills linked to interprofessional collaboration |
| 3. Behavioural change | Identifies individuals' transfer of interprofessional learning to their practice setting and their changed professional practice |
| 4a. Change in organisational practice | Wider changes in the organisation and delivery of care |
| 4b. Benefits to patients/clients | Improvements in health or wellbeing of patients/clients |

## The need for recognition and accreditation

Different actors formulate the need for interprofessional competences in health and social care, even after 30 years since the report of WHO (1988). The number of higher education institutions that implement course units explicitly focused on these competences remains scarce. Even in study programmes that have incorporated such course units the study volume devoted to the acquisition of interprofessional competences generally remains limited to about 1,5% of the total study volume (e.g., 2 or 3 ECTS credits out of 180). Some institutions or faculties incorporate a course unit to show that attention is given to this need, but fail to effectuate the acquisition of IP competences by students. Not only learning outcomes need to be formulated but also effective assessment needs to be organised.

As the EIPEN charter for IPE in Europe suggests, governmental agencies could focus on the compliance of clinical and educational institutions with regulations promoting and necessitating interprofessional practice and education, and should support the institutions by implementing accreditation and financial mechanisms that foster this practice and education. Professional bodies and quality assurance agencies also can incorporate interprofessional requirements in their frameworks for accrediting programmes or modules. EIPEN as a European Network may help in collaborating across borders, in order to strengthen the quality of interprofessional course units and study programmes, in higher education as well as in vocational education and training.

## Literature

Barr H (2000). Working together to learn together: Learning together to work together. *Journal of Interprofessional Care, 14*, 177–179.

Hammick M, Freeth D, Koppel I, Reebs S, & Barr H (2007). A best evidence systematic review of interprofessional education. *Medical Teacher, 29*, 735-751.

Kirkpatrick D (1967). Evaluation of training. In R Craig & L Bittel (Eds.), *Training and development handbook* (pp. 131-167). New York: McGraw-Hill.

Vyt A (2008). Interprofessional and transdisciplinary teamwork in health care. *Diabetes/Metabolism Research and Reviews, 24*, S106-S109.

Vyt A (2009). *Exploring quality assurance for interprofessional education in health and social care*. Antwerp/Apeldoorn: Garant Publishers.

Vyt A (2012). *Interprofessioneel en interdisciplinair samenwerken in gezondheid en welzijn [Interprofessional collaboration in health and social care]*. Antwerp/Apeldoorn: Garant-publishers.

Vyt A (2015). Interprofessional education and collaborative practice in health and social care: The need for transdisciplinary mindsets, instruments and mechanisms. In P Gibbs (Ed.), *Transdisciplinary professional learning and practice* (pp.69-88). Heidelberg/Zug: Springer Publishers.

World Health Organisation (1988). *Learning together to work together for health*. Technical Report Series No. 769. Geneva: WHO.

World Health Organisation (2010). *Framework for action on interprofessional education & collaborative practice*. Geneva: WHO.

World Health Organisation (2015). *Global strategy on people-centred and integrated health services*. Geneva: WHO

# Everyone benefits: Interprofessional work placement

Karin van Beek, Ivo Hendriks, Wietske Kuijer-Siebelink, Menno Pistorius and Marjolein Thijssen

HAN University of Applied Sciences promotes and facilitates cooperation between health care organisations, research institutions, and its departments focused on teaching and training. The global aim is to optimize health care. Work placement organisations combine education, research, and on-the-job training. Students, researchers and professionals work together intensively in interdisciplinary health care services and ongoing lines of research, while learning from each other throughout the process. They collectively develop new knowledge and insights that enrich the professionals' experience and vocational education. The topics of research are integrated rehabilitation care, prevention, diagnostics, treatment close to home, and e-health. Education and research programmes at the ZZG Herstelhotel Recovery and Rehabilitation Home focus on geriatric rehabilitation. Education and research programmes at the Thermion Academic Health Care Centre focus on cooperation in informal care and primary health care. There is also collaboration with hospitals.

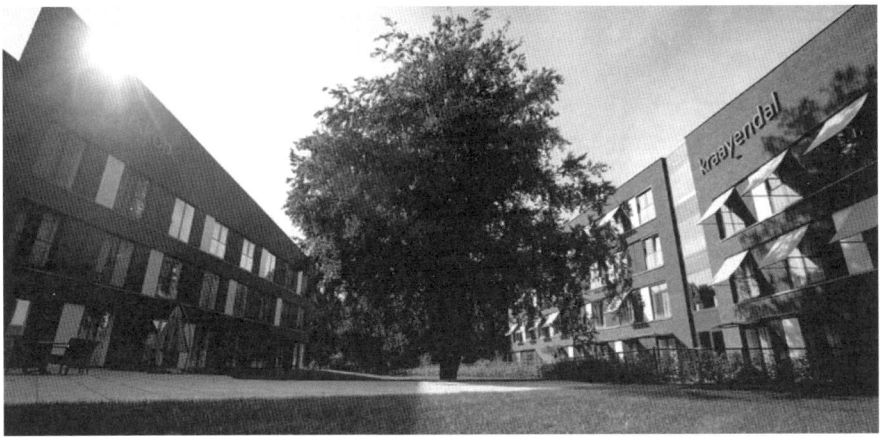

The Herstelhotel rehabilitation home, surrounded by woods.

## ZZG Herstelhotel

We are attending a multidisciplinary meeting at the Herstelhotel rehabilitation home. Sixteen students and two professionals are gathered round a large conference table. Process supporter Marianne has taken charge of the gathering. She draws everyone's attention to dietician Marelle, who is here today to offer the team nutritional support. The subject is the care plan for one of the patients. While the students are enjoying their cake – two of them are celebrating their birthdays – they take turns offering a little input about the patient. Medical terms are thrown about. The lady is hemiplegic and is confined to a wheelchair. She also suffers from constipation. "Does anyone have an idea why?" asks Marianne, the coordinator. A Nursing student thinks that it might be because she is not very mobile. Marianne wonders whether the tube feeding might also be part of the problem. The Nutrition and Dietetics students start thinking aloud. "Perhaps there isn't enough liquid in it, or perhaps the fibres are the cause." And while the students decorate their pieces of cake with M&Ms and whipped cream, dietician Marelle explains, "There are two types of fibre: one that ensures a soft consistency, and one that stimulates the peristaltic motion." And so the discussion continues. It moves on to the patient's level of functioning in everyday life. She can actually manage quite a lot. The students are unable to decide between levels two and three. "Let's say two and a half then", one of them muses. This comment is met with laughter, but the mood quickly turns serious again as the speech therapists start talking about the patient's swallowing therapy, apparently aimed at phasing out the tube feeding.

### Change agents

The ZZG Herstelhotel rehabilitation home, offering 180 beds, opened recently and is located in the woods between Groesbeek and Nijmegen. Patients who have undergone an operation or had a stroke, for example, come here to rehabilitate. Although it is in every way a rehabilitation centre, the brand new premises have something of the air of a hotel too, with a restaurant and a large patio. And the setting is simply amazing: wooded hills stretching far beyond the border into Germany. There are 150 people working at the Herstelhotel. The thirty HAN students are based in a separate room with a large conference table in the middle, surrounded by worktables holding computers and laptops. Ivo Hendriks, project manager for Quick and Optimal Recovery, the centre of expertise that organises the work placements, is proud of the place: "The word from the work floor is that students are a driving force for the organisation. They ask critical questions. This impacts the professionalism of the place. Change agents, we call them." That is partly because there is a large group of them working here together. "We have at least two students from each course. There's safety in numbers, and having a buddy also means you have a sparring partner to discuss things with."

## Multi

It is break time at the Herstelhotel. While the two occupational therapists start setting out wheelchairs for their clinical class, Sensor talks to some of the students. They are particularly full of praise for the multidisciplinary cooperation. A Nursing student offers an example: "Everyone is working together to treat a patient. The occupational therapists teach the patients how to dress themselves. We can then use that in nursing. This is a better approach, particularly in a rehabilitation setting. There's an informal atmosphere. We also teach clinical classes to each other. We'll be presenting our quality care project here, about catheterisation or contact isolation: how to treat someone with a serious bacterial infection." One of the Nutrition and Dietetics students is in her fourth year. She has the option of doing her graduation research here too. "I'm not actually sure whether I like the research here enough,' she says candidly. 'The project is looking at how protein-enriched bread impacts rehabilitation. I'd like to work with a different type of patient for a change."

## Team reflection

Inge and Marianne are the process coordinators for Herstelhotel, HAN lecturers Yvonne van de Wiel and Hans Joosten do the same for HAN. They join the students after the break for the team reflection. Yvonne takes charge: "This morning you began defining your goals. Let's talk about that." She goes down the list. Someone mentions having three evening shifts in a row. "One patient is receiving terminal care. I've never experienced a patient dying before. Yesterday I looked up what this will involve." Apparently it is not common for patients to die here, despite having an average age of eighty. All the students share what they are experiencing and what their goals are, until one student says, "What I really expect from a team reflection is that we talk about how we should work together." The discussion turns to the team reflection, to working together and to communication. The students do not just work together in a multidisciplinary setting, they also spend a lot of time sharing ideas about how to put this into practice together.

## Research

Herstelhotel is also a place of research. Thirteen students are spending half a year here doing research. Postdoctoral researcher Jaap Brunnekreef coordinates the research projects for the Institute of Health Studies (IHS). Herstelhotel is the largest provider of research placements for HAN in the region. It's an attractive partner in a very good setting. The whole idea is to bring the workplace to school. All IHS students go on a research placement. "They're not allowed to suggest their own research proposals. Part of the reason is the workplace – people would go crazy from all the research questions – but quality is also a factor. Physiotherapy's accreditation revealed that practice-based research needed to be looked at, which is an issue across HAN. The decision has now been made to use on-going lines of research. Each project builds on the work of the previous one", Jaap explains. There are four research groups right now. The overall 'difficulty' of the patients at Herstelhotel should be seen as a challenge, project manager Ivo Hendriks believes. "Particularly in this day and age, when financial resources are limited, studies need to be conducted to show how best to use funds. Should you have one-on-one practice sessions in physiotherapy? Can't they be given in groups? How should we encourage people to practice by themselves? Those are questions we want to ask."

## Exercise

A group of three students are researching how much patients exercise during therapy and outside. The students want to know whether the Herstelhotel setting ('a healing setting', the rehabilitation home's website proudly claims) is sufficiently inviting for exercise. Their research question concerns the activities that patients perform in addition to the scheduled therapy sessions, and how much time they spend on those activities. "On the one hand it's located in the middle of the woods, but on the other it's kind of hilly too," explains Aniek, one of the three students working on the project. "The idea is that the patients take walks, either by themselves, in groups or with their visitors. The vision is that Herstelhotel's surroundings invite people to exercise. We're trying to find out whether this is explained during therapy." The students' research involves conducting interviews and asking patients to keep daily activity records. They also want to take a look during physiotherapy sessions, with stopwatches at the ready, to see how much time the patients actually spend exercising. In September the students began drawing up a plan of action. "We're still waiting for a tool from Australia, where a score chart was developed for a similar research project." The groups are also looking for literature on the standards for how much exercise patients should be getting. When their research is complete, the next group will define a new research question, for example, how to entice patients to exercise more.

## On a roll

We return to the multidisciplinary team. Some of the students will return to their departments after this session, but first there is a clinical class about wheelchairs. Today it is the turn of Kim and Sanne, Occupational Therapy students. They begin by handing out evaluation forms. During the class the students are asked to record the level at which they believe that the two have mastered skills like presenting information. As it turns out every little part of a wheelchair has been carefully considered, enabling every chair to be tailored exactly to suit each patient. "Here we have some of the most frequently used wheelchairs", they announce. "This is a semi-active one, for both hand and foot propulsion." Kim asks the audience what their experiences are. That leads them back to this morning's patient. Sanne explains how her wheelchair has been completely geared to accommodate her hemiplegia. Finally the time comes to take a ride in those chairs: no talking, just laughing, pushing and pulling.

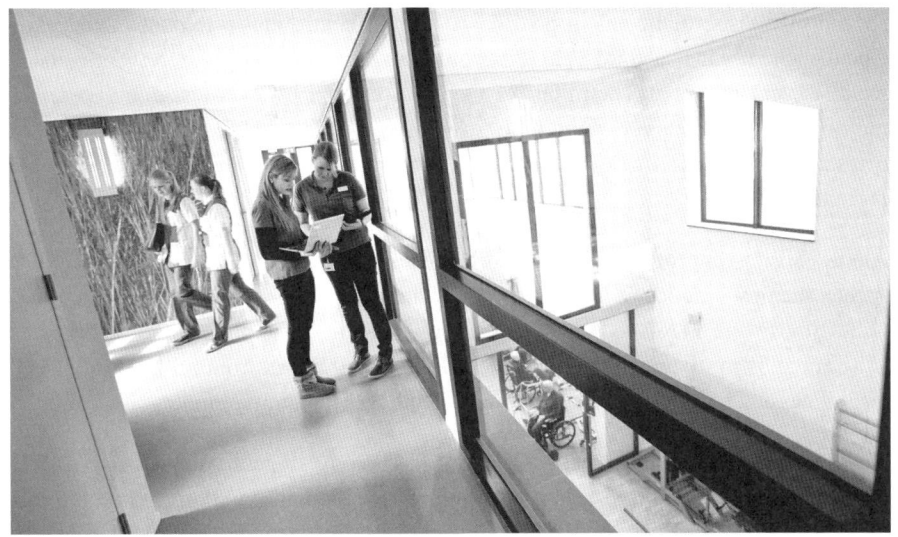

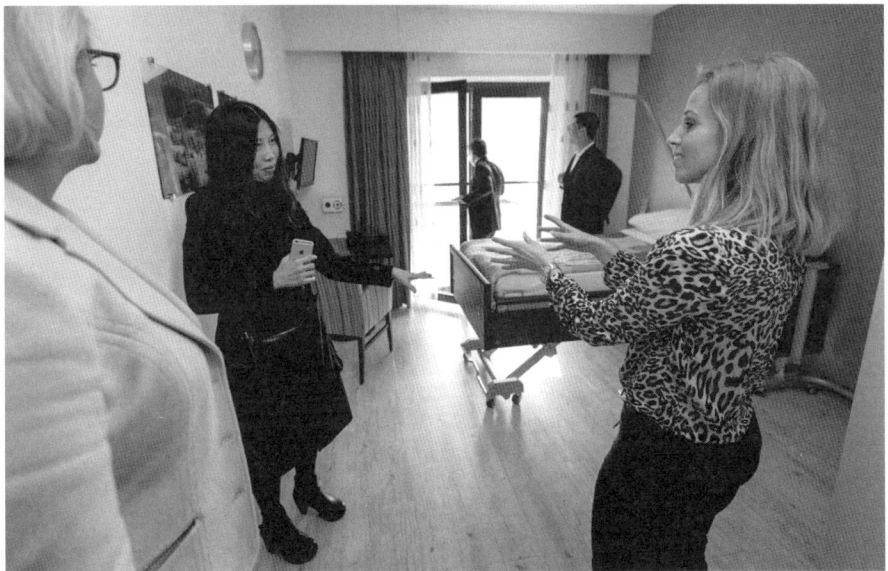

Students and process coordinators at Herstelhotel and HAN work together in a multidisciplinary setting.

## Academic Health Care Centre Thermion

Academic Health Care Centre Thermion in Waalsprong, built on the beautifully renovated premises that once housed a Philips factory, is the result of a partnership between the Radboud UMC and a series of primary health care providers such as a general medical practice, a dental practice, a physiotherapy practice, psychologists, speech therapists, dieticians, a pharmacy, a child centre and a ParkinsonNet team. Claudia Graafmans, a third-year Physiotherapy student doing her research placement, is very happy at Thermion. "This is a great place to do research. There are multiple project groups working here, so you always have someone to talk to if you get stuck. Or you can go directly to the professionals at Thermion if you have a question."

Aukje Zijlstra, one of the third-year students doing her first work placement at a speech therapy practice at the centre, agrees that Thermion is a great place to work. "The atmosphere is relaxed, and interacting with other disciplines in the workplace is a source of motivation. The weekly meetings of trainees from all the established disciplines at Thermion provide a more in-depth understanding of integrated care."

Niels Hennekam, a fourth-year Occupational Therapy student conducting practice-based research on the preferences and needs of people with multimorbidity in terms of integrated care, describes the people involved as "accessible and enthusiastic", even though he is not always overly happy with the day-to-day practice. "The work itself can be a bit boring: a lot of time at the computer, a lot of theory." Yet all the students see Thermion as a challenging place to work. "It's challenging in that it's still a new concept, where people are open to new ideas and research", says Renske Seves, a fourth-year Occupational Therapy student who is also doing research on client perspectives. It has given her a boost in her professionalism. "Being approached in this way feels like you're almost a professional yourself."

## Improvement

Yvette Beulen, fourth-year Nutrition and Dietetics student who is doing the same practice-based research as her colleagues Niels and Renske, has more experience with multidisciplinary work placements: she previously did a work placement at the ZZG Herstelhotel rehabilitation home, and perhaps as a result has a more critical view of this type of work placement. "I'm definitely a supporter of this setting. You learn to look beyond the confines of your own field and to see and utilise the qualities that others possess." Yet she still sees room for improvement. "People will probably learn more if more meetings are organised for the 'regular' and research trainees together. At Herstelhotel, we already saw something of a division between the two groups, and sadly the same is true here. It's a little disappointing to see how little communication and knowledge sharing there is between trainees and regular staff."

Her colleague Renske Seves agrees: "If more of those meetings were organised, the trainees would be more involved in the research and the researchers would have a better idea of what's happening in the workplace. They could approach each other with questions and complement each other. Now they sometimes both work separately on the same thing, which is a pity."

Speech Therapy trainee Aukje, however, is not surprised there is still room for improvement: "This is the second half year the work placement project has been up and running, and occasionally it's still unclear what the best approach is. But things are well organised and there's definitely no lack of clarity or structure, and I feel that the meetings are utilised well. A great deal of effort, attention and time goes into them in a useful and educational manner."

## Professional practice

Despite her criticism of how research students and trainees work together, Renske is impressed by the interpersonal dealings at Thermion. "People all treat each other as equals: the doctors, the paramedical disciplines and the students. The practitioners drop by for a chat. This leads to new contacts that could be valuable for our research." Those contacts are not only useful: the students believe that working together like this closely reflects the professional practice. Aukje is in fact convinced the multidisciplinary character is a necessary element: "I've seen how I will be expected to work as a speech therapist at a care centre. Without this work placement I'd only have studied monodisciplinary care." Aukje believes this link is very important in this day and age: "Yes, considering the changes in the health care sector. The expectations that insurers have of practitioners are changing, partly as costs are being cut everywhere. To improve efficiency in care, the separate disciplines need to step beyond their individual borders. You need to understand your colleagues' profession to make better referrals." Niels also appreciates this understanding of other disciplines: "I now know what disciplines are involved with chronically sick patients, for example. This is very interesting for me as a future occupational therapist." Yvette also applies the lessons to her own situation: "These experiences have taught me that I should aim for integrated multidisciplinary care in my professional practice."

Clearly, despite the few points of criticism, the students are enthusiastic about their placement projects at Thermion. At the same time, of course, the students bring something to the table too. For example, Claudia's research will map out the needs of the residents of Lent in terms of physical therapies. Thermion will use her findings to better gear that care to the residents, which benefits everyone in the end.

## Acknowledgements

This chapter was also written with input from Aukje Zijlstra (work placement, third-year Speech Therapy), Claudia Graafmans (practice-based research, third-year Physiotherapy), Yvette Beulen (practice-based research, fourth-year Nutrition and Dietetics), Renske Seves (practice-based research, fourth-year Occupational Therapy), and Niels Hennekam (practice-based research, fourth-year Occupational Therapy).

# Epilogue

We have come to the end of a journey through some policy issues and a variety of European examples of good practice in interprofessional education. Contributions in this book have been written by academics from institutional members of the European Interprofessional Practice and Education Network (EIPEN).

Interprofessional education has gained interest in the past decades, but is still underdeveloped. Isolated initiatives from universities and higher education institutions are not sufficient to meet the needs and challenges of high-quality health care in which collaborative practice is perceived as an essential component.

Like in Canada, Australia, and the USA, a network of institutions can give an impetus to develop an interprofessional culture not only in higher education but also in clinical practice. Joint forces are needed on regional, national, and European level. Interprofessionalism can help in making health and social care more patient-centred but also more adequate, efficient and cost-effective.

Within Europe, the Nordic countries and the UK have been pioneering in creating interprofessional courses, also stimulated by governmental policies and health care authorities. EIPEN acts as an umbrella organisation, linking European institutions and regional networks, creating a forum for exchange between academics, clinicians and policymakers. An open interprofessional culture, with highly competent health care professionals in collaborative practice, is needed to develop and deploy an efficient and a sustainable health care system. Let us hope for a gradual evolution moving from "some interesting initiatives in some European countries" towards a real pan-European area of interprofessional education and collaborative practice.

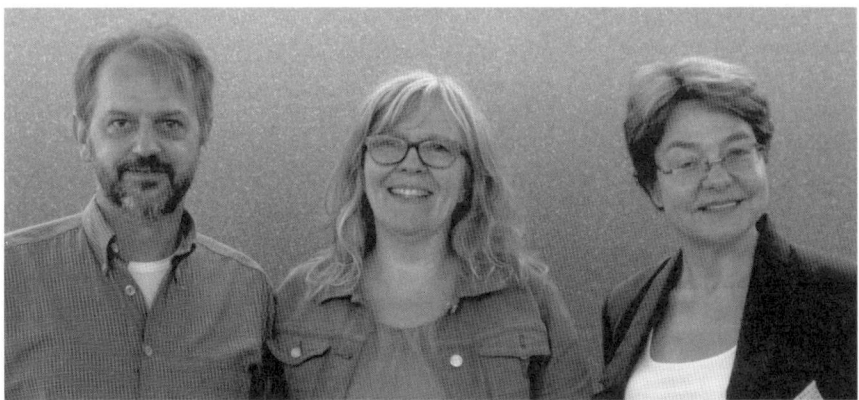

The editors of this book, wishing IPE to be implemented all over Europe.

For information on interprofessional practice and education in Europe, visit the website of the European Interprofessional Practice and Education Network (EIPEN):

www.eipen.eu